THE NEW ZERO POINT WEIGHT LOSS COOKBOOK

50 + Delicious Recipes for Every Meal to Help You Lose Weight and Stay Healthy | Includes 20-Day Meal Plan and Full-Color Photos

Diane Dobbins

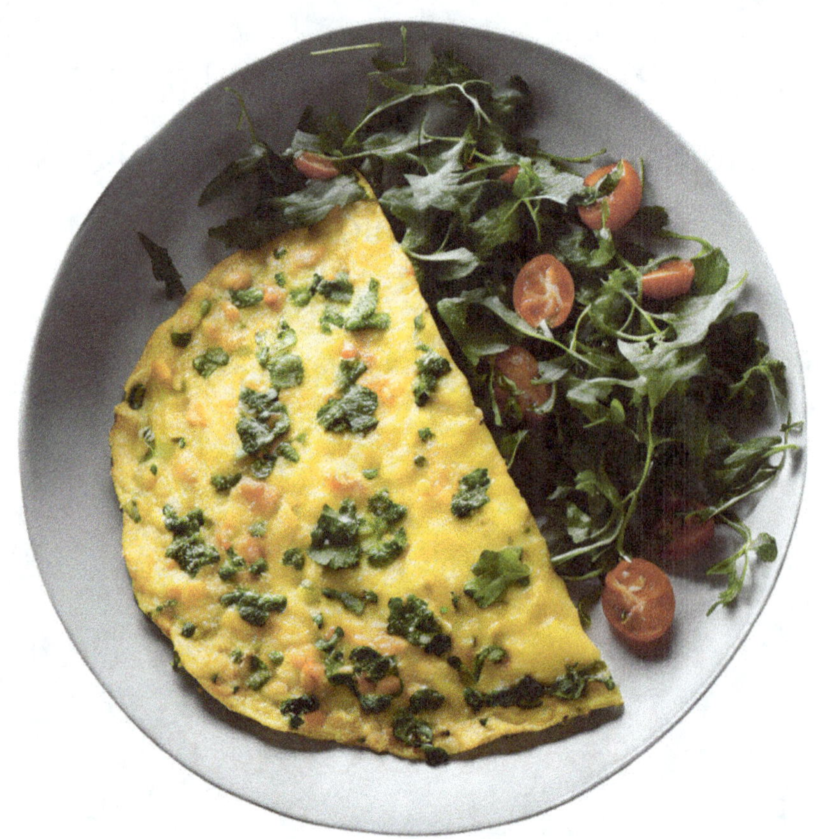

TABLE OF CONTENT

Introduction 5

The Science Behind Zero Point Foods 5

How to Use This Cookbook 6

Chapter 1: Zero Point Concept 7

Change in Behavior 7

What Makes Food Zero-Point 7

Nutritional Density 7

Low Density of Calories 7

Satiety 7

The Benefits of Incorporating Zero Point Foods 8

Overall Health Benefits 8

Examples of Zero Point Foods 9

Examples of Non-Zero Point Foods 10

Caloric Needed for Weight Loss 10

Applying This to a Zero-Point Diet 11

Chapter 2 Breakfast recipes 13

Veggie Omelette 14

Fruit and Yogurt Parfait 15

Spinach and Mushroom Scramble 16

Banana Pancakes 17

Berry Smoothie Bowl 18

Apple Pie Parfait 19

4Ingredient Microwave Mug Frittata 20

Salmon Omelet in a Mug 21

Skinny Western Omelet Muffins 22

Kodiak Cake Muffins 23

Cheesy Ham and Egg Cups 24

W.W. Crepes 24

Chapter 3 lunch recipes 25

 Grilled Chicken Salad 26

Vegetable StirFry 27

Turkey Lettuce Wraps 28

Quinoa and Black Bean Salad 29

Cucumber and Tomato Salad 30

Chipotle Chicken Casserole 31

Grilled Crab Legs 32

Baked Zucchini Chips 33

Jello Grapes 34

Lemon Greek Chicken Skewers 35

Egg Salad 36

One Pan Chicken Fajitas 37

3Bean Turkey Chili 38

Chicken Enchilada Stuffed Zucchini 39

Buffalo Chicken Lettuce Wraps 40

Chapter 4 dinner recipes 41

 Baked Salmon with Asparagus 42

Zucchini Noodles with Marinara Sauce 43

Chicken and Vegetable Skewers 44

Stuffed Bell Peppers 45

Cauliflower Fried Rice 46

Slow Cooker Tomato Balsamic Chicken 47

Turkey, Corn, and Black Bean Chili 48

Lentil Soup 49

Garden Vegetable Soup 50

Crockpot Bean Soup — 51

Slow Cooker Tuscan Lentil Sloppy Joes — 52

Cabbage Soup — 53

Instant Pot Vegetarian Chili — 54

Skinny Bang Bang Shrimp — 55

Grilled Shrimp Marinade with Shrimp Sauce — 56

Chapter 5 Apple Slices with Cinnamon — 57

Carrot and Celery Sticks with Hummus — 59

HardBoiled Eggs — 60

Cucumber Slices with Greek Yogurt Dip — 62

Frozen Fruit Pops — 63

Spicy Roasted Cauliflower — 64

Weight Watchers Cheesecake — 65

Mango Corn Salsa — 76

Slow Cooker Spaghetti Squash — 67

Slow Cooker Tomato Sauce — 68

Smiley's Famous Zero Point B.B.Q. Sauce — 69

Bonus — 71

Conclusion — 75

INTRODUCTION

Are you tired of restrictive diets that leave you feeling hungry and deprived? Have you struggled with yo-yo dieting, only to find yourself back where you started or worse off? You're not alone. Many people face these challenges in their weight loss journey. This book addresses these pain points and provides a sustainable, enjoyable way to achieve your health and weight loss goals.

the Zero Point Weight Loss Recipes Cookbook is your ultimate guide to a healthier lifestyle through the principles of the Weight Watchers (W.W.) zero-point food system. This approach emphasizes foods low in calories but high in nutritional value, allowing you to eat satisfying meals without the constant stress of counting points or calories.

Foods designated as zero points are chosen for their general health benefits, satiety value, and nutritional density. Usually low in bad fats and carbohydrates, these meals contain vitamins, minerals, fiber, and lean protein. The premise is that you can naturally control your appetite and energy intake by prioritizing certain items, which may reduce weight and increase your health.

1. Nutritional Density: Compared to their calorie level, nutritionally rich foods provide a high concentration of vital nutrients. For instance, low in calories yet high in vitamins, minerals, and fiber include leafy greens, vegetables, fruits, and lean meats. This makes them great options for satisfying your hunger without exceeding your daily caloric intake.

2. Satiety Value: Satiation is the sensation of fullness and contentment after a meal. Because they keep you fuller for longer, meals high in satiation may help regulate appetite and lower total calorie consumption. Because they effectively promote satiety, meals high in protein, like chicken, turkey, and fish, and fiber, such as beans, lentils, and vegetables, are essential components of zero-point foods.

3. Health Benefits: Zero-point items are selected for their favorable effects on general health and their ability to help with weight reduction. Consuming these foods may lower your chance of developing long-term conditions, including diabetes, heart disease, and certain types of cancer. Fruits and vegetables, for instance, are rich in antioxidants that help the body fight inflammation and oxidative stress.

This cookbook serves as your all-inclusive manual for preparing and savoring zero-point foods. Every chapter covers a variety of meals, including breakfast, lunch, supper, and snacks and sweets. Here's how to use this cookbook to its fullest:

1. Start with the Basics: Learn about the meals on the list that have no points and why they suit you. You can prepare balanced meals and make wise decisions with this information.

2. Explore the Recipes: Every dish in this cookbook has been thoughtfully created to be tasty, simple, and consistent with the zero-point concept. There are many alternatives to fit your likes and preferences, from filling meals to robust brunches
.

3. Plan Your Meals: Using the 20-day meal plan as a template to organize your eating. You can remain on track and avoid harmful last-minute decisions by organizing your meals in advance.

4. Customize and Experiment: You can alter the recipes to your preference. Make these dishes your own by adding your favorite zero-point items and experimenting with various flavors. Because zero-point items are so versatile, you can get creative and customize meals in the kitchen.

5. Enjoy the Journey: Accept the zero-point path as a constructive way of life. Consider the advantages of consuming wholesome meals, and enjoy the experience of trying out different dishes and tastes.

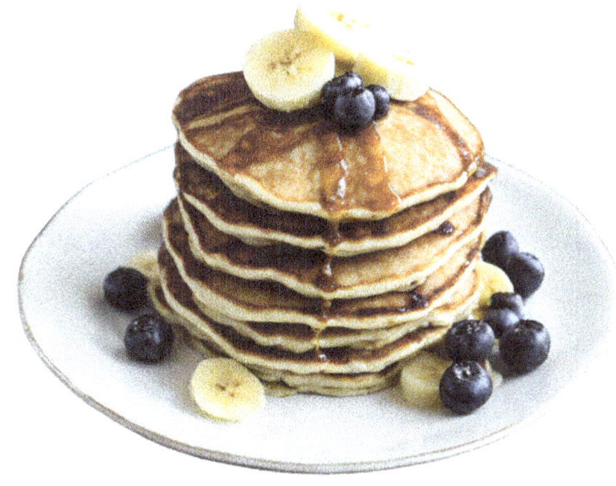

Chapter 1: Zero Point Concept

The concept of zero points in the context of the Weight Watchers program is also a transformative approach to weight loss and healthy eating. It is intended to make tracking one's food intake easier while encouraging nutrient-dense meals that help weight control and general wellness. Foods marked as zero points may be freely consumed without careful monitoring, promoting the development of healthy eating habits and maintaining a sustainable diet.

Why Zero Points food?

The main goal of zero-point foods is to promote the eating of complete, unprocessed foods that are naturally rich in vital nutrients yet low in calories. These meals have been chosen for their capacity to satisfy hunger, control it, and provide several health advantages without adding a substantial amount of calories to daily consumption. People may still reach their weight reduction objectives while enjoying a varied and fulfilling diet by concentrating on zero-point meals.

- ### Change in Behavior

The zero-point system signifies a substantial change in eating habits. Conventional calorie counting is time-consuming and often causes dissatisfaction and fatigue. On the other hand, the zero-point system provides a more adaptable and straightforward method, lessening the mental strain involved in meal monitoring. This change facilitates people's development of a more positive connection with food, seeing it as a source of sustenance instead of a collection of variables that need to be controlled.

What Makes Food Zero-Point?

Foods that meet many criteria that align with nutritional research and weight control concepts are designated zero-point foods. These standards include satiety, low-calorie density, nutritional density, and general health advantages. Let's examine each factor more detail to determine what constitutes a zero-point meal.

- ### Nutritional Density

The concentration of vital nutrients in the food's calorie content is called nutritional density. Zero-point meals are often high in fiber, vitamins, minerals, and lean proteins—all essential for sustaining body processes and preserving health. For instance, fruits and vegetables are low in calories but high in fiber, potassium, and vitamins C and A. Because of their excellent nutrient-to-calorie ratio, they are perfect to include as meals with no points.

-

The number of calories per unit weight of food is known as its calorie density. Foods with low-calorie density fill the stomach with substantial space while supplying fewer calories, aiding in satiety. Zero-point meals' substantial fiber and water content helps explain their low-calorie density. For example, leafy greens, non-starchy vegetables, and broth-based soups are low-calorie, satisfying alternatives that count toward your daily goal.

- Satiety

The fullness and pleasure following a meal help regulate appetite and lower total caloric intake. This is known as satiety. Foods high in satiation usually include fiber and protein, slowing digestion and extending the sensation of fullness. Lean proteins with high protein and fiber content, such as skinless chicken breast, turkey, fish, and lentils and beans, are essential items on the zero-point food list.

- Overall Health Benefits

Foods that are zero points are also picked because they are suitable for your general health. Consuming these foods may lower your chance of developing long-term conditions, including diabetes, heart disease, and certain types of cancer. Fruits and vegetables, for instance, are rich in antioxidants that help the body fight inflammation and oxidative stress. Lean proteins also assist in maintaining and rebuilding muscles, while fiber facilitates digestion and blood sugar regulation.

1. Sustainable Weight Loss: You may establish a calorie deficit without constantly monitoring your intake by prioritizing zero-point items. This method facilitates long-term weight reduction by simplifying and streamlining the process of eating healthily.

2. Nutritional Balance: Foods with zero points contribute to a diet rich in vital nutrients. This may result in increased vitality, better digestion, and overall well-being improvement.

3. Flexibility and Freedom: You may enjoy various meals without feeling deprived because of the zero-point system's flexibility and freedom. This might lessen the chance of overindulging or binge eating since you can always satiate your appetite with zero-point meals.

4. Improved Relationship with Food: You may create a more positive relationship with food by emphasizing whole, nourishing meals. You may enjoy food as a source of sustenance and pleasure rather than seeing it as the adversary.

Examples of Zero Point Foods

Here are some examples of zero-point meals and their advantages to help paint a better picture:

- Vegetables: The majority of non-starchy veggies have 0 points. This category includes Broccoli, spinach, carrots, tomatoes, and bell peppers. These veggies give dishes body without adding many calories and are rich in vitamins, minerals, and fiber.
- Fruits: Null points are awarded for fresh fruits such as apples, berries, oranges, and grapes. Fruits are naturally sweet and a good source of fiber, antioxidants, and vitamins C and A.
- Lean Proteins: Fish, shellfish, skinless chicken breast, and turkey breast are all zero points. These proteins are rich in protein and low in calories and fat, which keeps you feeling full and maintains the health of your muscles.
- Eggs: Eggs are 0 points and a great source of high-quality protein. They are adaptable and work well in various dishes, including breakfast and supper.
- Legumes: There are no points for beans, lentils, or peas. They are a filling and nourishing addition to your diet since they are rich in protein and fiber.
- Non-Fat Yogurt: Non-fat Greek and plain yogurt are worth 0 points. They help maintain healthy bones and muscles because they are excellent providers of calcium and protein.

Although the foundation of the W.W. program comprises zero-point items, it's crucial to understand which foods are not zero points because of their greater calorie density or poorer nutritional value. Here are a few items that don't count as 0 points:

- Processed Foods: Generally, foods heavy in harmful fats, added sugars, and processed grains are not zero points. This covers foods like chips, cookies, and sugar-filled cereals. These meals are high in calories and often deficient in essential nutrients.
- Starchy Vegetables: Although full of nutrients, starchy vegetables such as potatoes, maize, and peas are not zero points because of their greater calorie and carb content. When including them in your diet, portion management is essential.
- Full-Fat Dairy: Items high in fat, such as cheese, whole milk, and cream, do not count against your point total. They include more fat and calories, which, if ingested in excess, may cause weight gain.
- Red Meat: Because of their more excellent fat content, lean meats like pig and beef do not count as zero points in a balanced diet, even if they may be. Points may be managed by selecting leaner choices and paying attention to portion sizes.
- Grains and Bread: Whole grains, such as quinoa, brown rice, and whole-wheat bread, are low in calories but not fat. Because of their increased calorie and carb content, it's crucial to monitor quantities and ingest them carefully.

Caloric Needed for Weight Loss

To lose weight, however, paying attention to your total calorie intake is crucial—even while following a Zero Point diet. The scientific method used to calculate the ideal calorie intake for weight reduction is broken down as follows:

1. Basal Metabolic Rate (B.M.R.)
B.M.R. represents the calories your body needs to maintain essential physiological functions like breathing, circulation, and cell production while at rest. The B.M.R. can be estimated using the Harris-Benedict equation:
For men: $BMR = 88.362 + (13.397 \times \text{weight in kg}) + (4.799 \times \text{height in cm}) - (5.677 \times \text{age in years})$

- For women BMR = 447.593 + (9.247 \times \text{weight in kg}) + (3.098 \times \text{height in cm}) – (4.330 \times \text{age in years})

2. Total Daily Energy Expenditure (T.D.E.E.)

T.D.E.E. includes B.M.R. plus additional calories burned through physical activity. T.D.E.E. is calculated by multiplying the B.M.R. by an activity factor:
- Sedentary (little or no exercise): B.M.R. (times) 1.2
- Lightly active (light exercise/sports 1-3 days/week): B.M.R. (times) 1.375
- Moderately active (moderate exercise/sports 3-5 days/week): B.M.R. (times) 1.55
- Very active (hard exercise/sports 6-7 days a week): B.M.R. (times) 1.725
- Super active (tough exercise/sports & physical job or 2x training): B.M.R. (times) 1.9

3. Caloric Deficit for Weight Loss

To lose weight, a caloric deficit is needed. A standard recommendation is to reduce daily caloric intake by 500-1000 calories, leading to a weight loss of approximately 0.5 to 1 kg (1 to 2 pounds) per week.

Example Calculation

Let's consider an example of a 35-year-old man who weighs 70 kg and is 165 cm tall, with a moderately active lifestyle:

1. Calculate BMR: BMR = 447.593 + (9.247 \times 70) + (3.098 \times 165) – (4.330 \times 35) = 447.593 + 647.29 + 511.17 – 151.55 = 1454.503
2. Calculate TDEE: TDEE = BMR \times 1.55 = 1454.503 \times 1.55 = 2254.48
3. Caloric Deficit: For weight loss, she might aim for a daily caloric intake of 2254.48 – 500 = 1754.48 \text{ calories/day}

Applying This to a Zero-Point Diet

Even though Zero Point meals are meant to be nutrient-dense and low in calories, monitoring your total caloric intake is essential. The user should ensure that most of their diet comprises ZeroPoint items and strive for the calorie consumption determined above. This strategy encourages satiety and nourishment while assisting in maintaining the calorie deficit required for weight reduction.

- Track overall intake: Even with Zero Point foods, tracking total caloric intake is essential, especially when consuming non-Zero Point foods.
- Balance meals: Include various foods to ensure adequate intake of all essential nutrients.
- Listen to your body: Eat when hungry and stop when complete, using Zero Point foods to manage hunger without exceeding caloric needs.

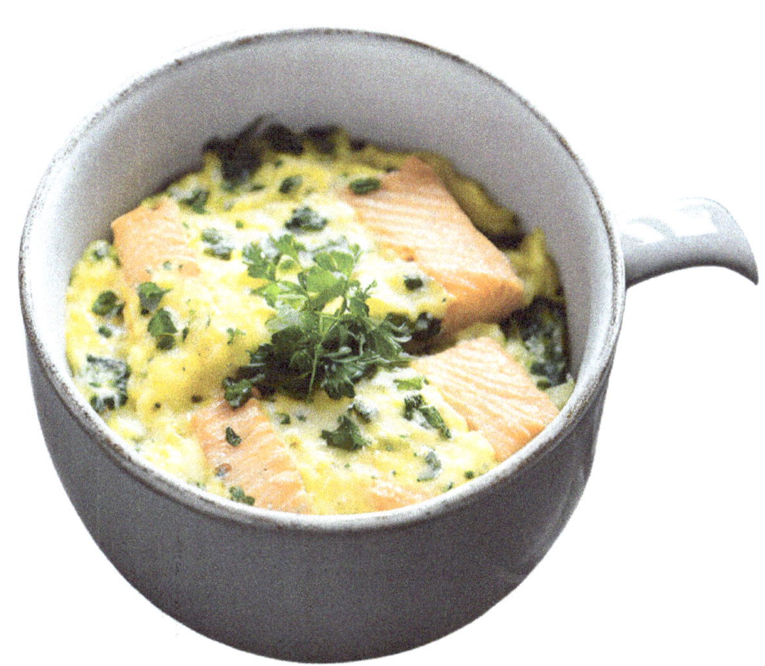

CHAPTER TWO

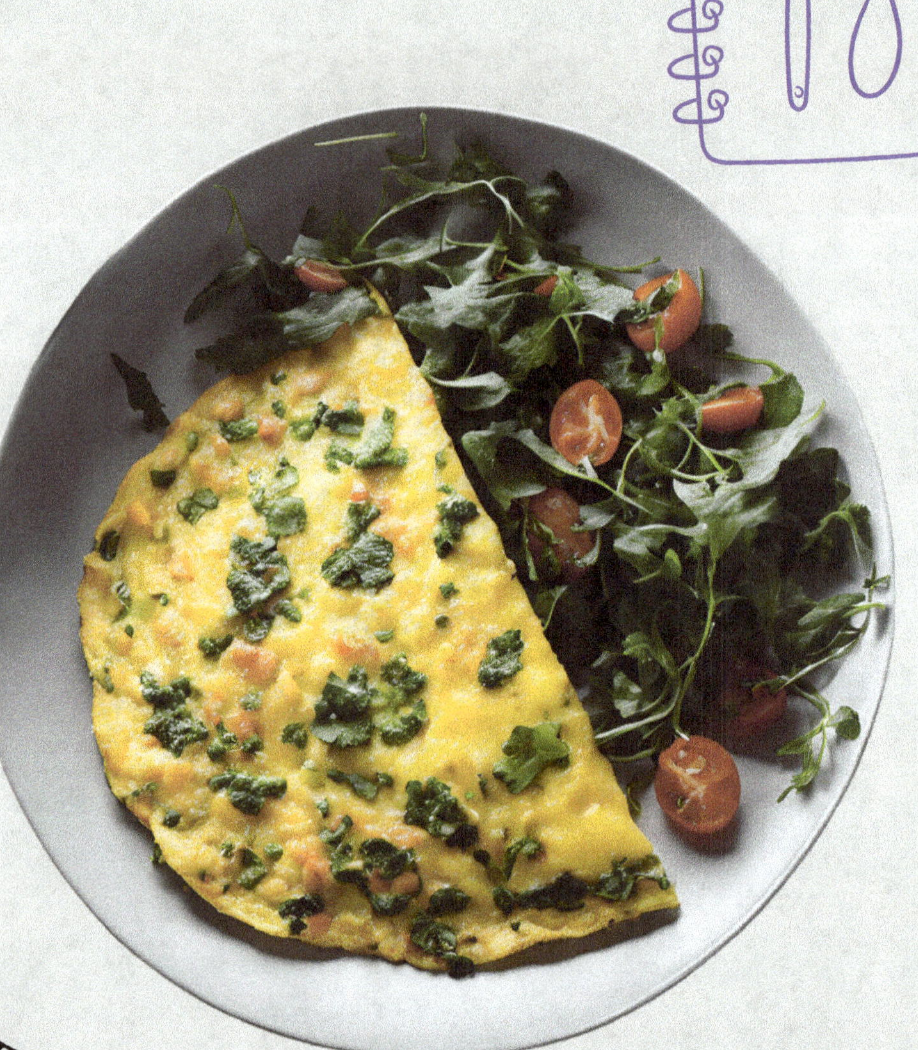

Breakfast Recipes

Veggie Omelette

Brighten your morning with colorful Veggie Omelets, a low-calorie, nutrient-packed breakfast that will keep you full and satisfied.

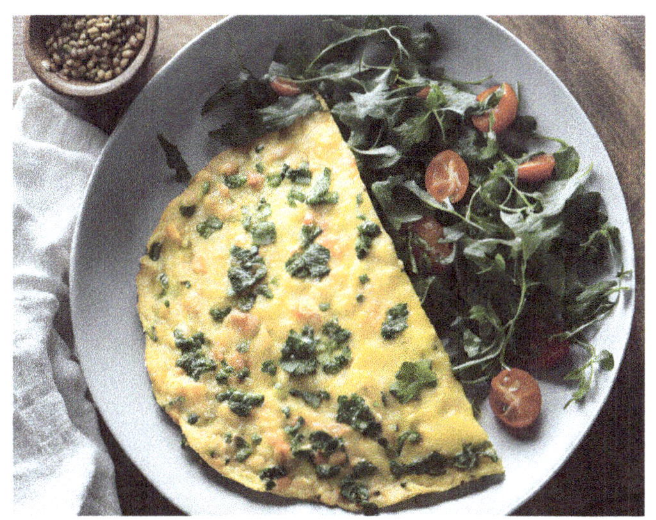

ingredients

- 1 cup egg whites
- 1/2 cup chopped bell peppers (red, green, yellow)
- 1/4 cup chopped onions
- 1/4 cup chopped tomatoes

- 1/4 cup chop2ped Spinach
- Salt and pepper to taste
- Fresh herbs (optional, for garnish)

Preparation Time

4-5 minutes per pancake

Serving Size

Makes about 12 pancakes

Nutrition (per serving)

Calories: 140 Protein: 12g
Carbohydrates: 6g Fiber:2g
Fat: 8g

Instructions

1. Prepare the Vegetables: Chop all your vegetables and set them aside.

2. Cook the Vegetables: In a nonstick skillet, sauté the bell peppers, onions, and tomatoes over medium heat until tender, about 34 minutes.

3. Add Spinach: Add the spinach and cook until it is wilted, for about 1 minute.

4. Pour Egg Whites: Pour the egg whites over the cooked vegetables and season with salt and pepper. Cook until the egg whites are set, about 34 minutes.

5. Fold and Serve: Gently fold the omelet in half and slide it onto a plate. Garnish with fresh herbs if desired.

Fruit and Yogurt Parfait

Treat yourself to a refreshing Fruit and Yogurt Parfait. This delightful mix of creamy yogurt and fresh berries is zero points and a delicious way to fuel your morning.

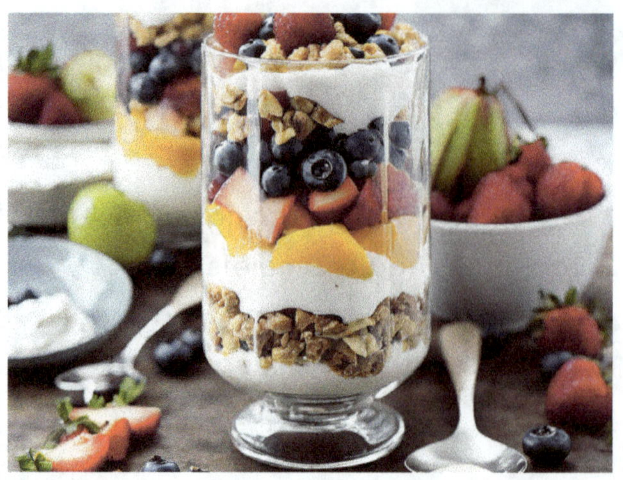

ingredients

- 1 cup fatfree Greek yogurt
- 1/2 cup mixed berries (strawberries, blueberries, raspberries)
- 1 tablespoon zeropoint granola (optional)
- 1 teaspoon honey (optional)

Preparation Time
Total Time: 5 minutes

Cooking Time
None

Serving Size
1

Nutrition (per serving)
- Protein: 10g
- Carbs: 12g
- Fat: 0g

Instructions

1. Layer the Yogurt: In a tall glass or parfait dish, spoon a layer of Greek yogurt.

2. Add Berries: Add a layer of mixed berries to the yogurt.

3. Repeat Layers: Repeat the layers until all ingredients are used, finishing with a layer of berries.

4. Top It Off: Sprinkle with zeropoint granola and drizzle with honey if desired.

Spinach and Mushroom Scramble

Elevate your breakfast game with this Spinach and Mushroom Scramble. It's a savory and hearty meal that packs a punch of flavor while keeping your calorie count in check.

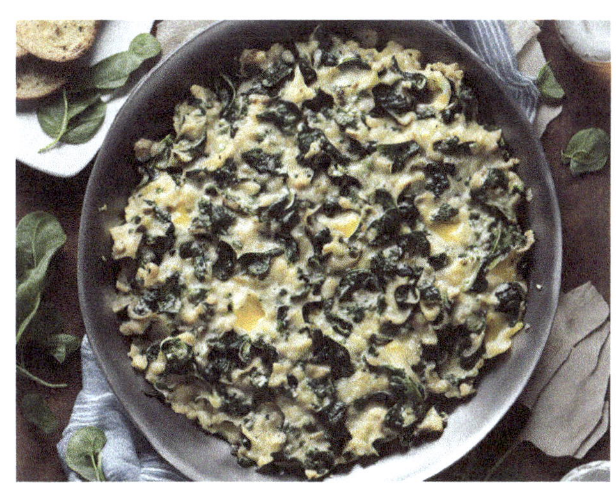

ingredients

- 1 cup egg whites
- 1/2 cup sliced mushrooms
- 1 cup fresh spinach
- 1/4 cup diced onions
- Salt and pepper to taste

Preparation Time

Total Time: 10 minutes

Cooking Time

7 minutes

Serving Size

1

Nutrition (per serving)

- Protein: 15g
- Carbs: 4g
- Fat: 0g

Instructions

1. Cook Onions and Mushrooms: In a nonstick skillet, sauté the onions and mushrooms over medium heat until tender, about 5 minutes.

2. Add Spinach: Add the spinach and cook until it is wilted, for about 1 minute.

3. Add Egg Whites: Pour in the egg whites and season with salt and pepper. Cook, stirring frequently, until the eggs are fully cooked, about 34 minutes.

4. Serve: Serve immediately.

Banana Pancakes

Enjoy the natural sweetness of bananas with these easy Banana Pancakes. These fluffy pancakes are perfect for a quick and healthy breakfast that feels like a treat.

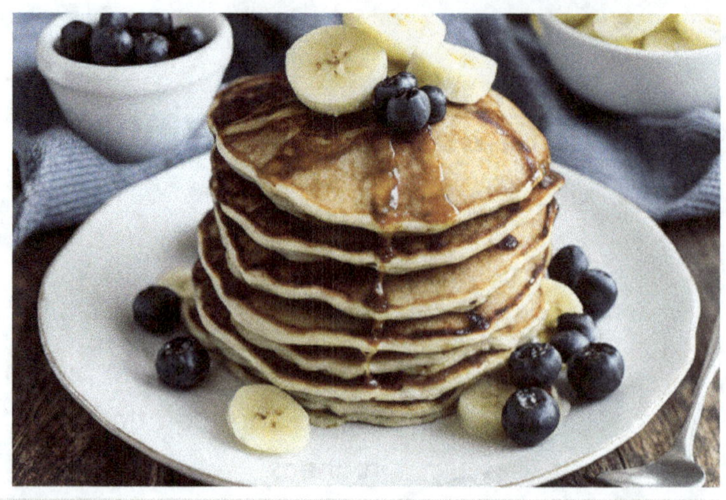

ingredients

- 1 ripe banana
- 2 eggs
- 1/4 teaspoon baking powder
- 1/2 teaspoon vanilla extract
- Pinch of cinnamon

Preparation Time

Total Time: 10 minutes

Cooking Time

5 minutes

Serving Size

1

Nutrition (per serving)

- Protein: 12g
- Carbs: 18g
- Fat: 2g

Instructions

1. Mash the Banana: In a bowl, mash the banana until smooth.

2. Mix Ingredients: Add the eggs, baking powder, vanilla extract, and cinnamon. Mix until well combined.

3. Cook Pancakes: Heat a nonstick skillet over medium heat. Pour small amounts of the Batter onto the skillet to form pancakes. Cook until bubbles form on the surface, then flip and cook until golden brown, about 2 minutes per side.

4. Serve: Serve warm.

Berry Smoothie Bowl

Start your day with a burst of freshness with this Berry Smoothie Bowl. Packed with antioxidants and vibrant colors, it's as nutritious as beautiful.

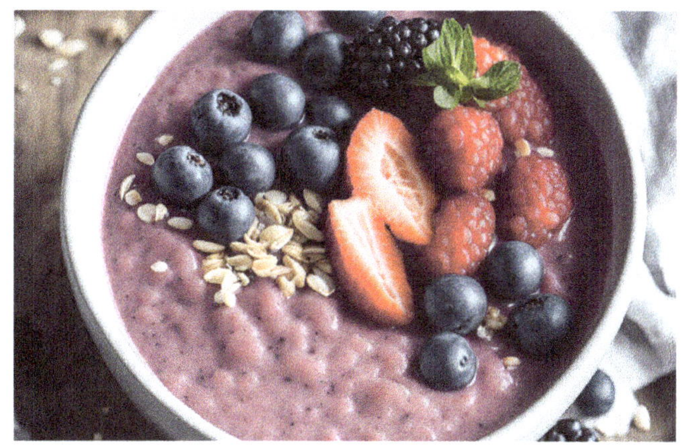

ingredients

- 1 cup frozen mixed berries
- 1/2 banana
- 1/2 cup fatfree Greek yogurt

- 1/4 cup unsweetened almond milk
- Toppings: fresh berries, sliced banana, granola (optional), chia seeds (optional)

Preparation Time
Total Time: 5 minutes

Cooking Time
None

Serving Size
1

Nutrition (per serving)
- Protein: 15g
- Carbs: 20g
- Fat: 0g

Instructions

1. Blend Ingredients: In a blender, combine the frozen berries, banana, Greek yogurt, and almond milk. Blend until smooth.

2. Pour and Top: Pour the smoothie into a bowl and top with fresh berries, sliced banana, granola, and chia seeds if desired.

Apple Pie Parfait

This Apple Pie Parfait gives you all the flavors of your favorite dessert in a healthy, zeropoint breakfast option. It's quick, delicious, and feels like an indulgence without the guilt!

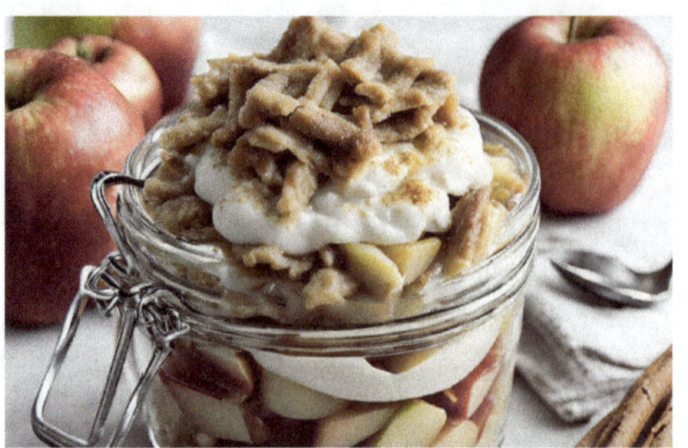

ingredients

- 1 cup fatfree Greek yogurt
- 1 apple, peeled, cored, and diced
- 1/2 teaspoon cinnamon
- 1/4 teaspoon nutmeg
- 1 tablespoon water
- 1 teaspoon zerocalorie sweetener (optional)
- 1 tablespoon zeropoint granola (optional)

Preparation Time

Total Time: 10 minutes

Cooking Time

None

Serving Size

1

Nutrition (per serving)

- Protein: 12g
- Carbs: 18g
- Fat: 0g

Instructions

1. Cook the Apples: In a small saucepan, combine the diced apple, cinnamon, nutmeg, water, and sweetener. Cook over medium heat until the apples are tender, about 57 minutes.

2. Layer the Parfait: In a glass or bowl, layer the Greek yogurt and cooked apples. Repeat layers if desired.

3. Top It Off: Sprinkle with zeropoint granola for added crunch.

Salmon Omelet in a Mug

Elevate your breakfast with this Salmon Omelet in a Mug. It's a luxurious and proteinrich meal that's quick to prepare, perfect for busy mornings.

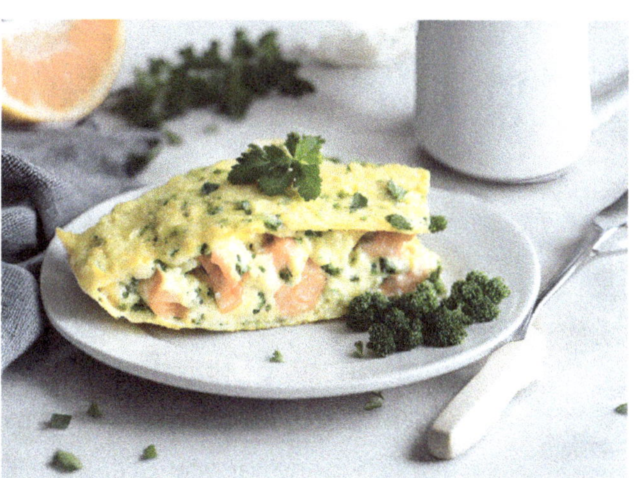

ingredients

- 1/2 cup egg whites
- 1/4 cup cooked salmon, flaked
- 1 tablespoon chopped green onions
- Salt and pepper to taste

Preparation Time

Total Time: 3 minutes

Cooking Time

2 minutes

Serving Size

1

Nutrition (per serving)

- Protein: 15g
- Carbs: 1g
- Fat: 2g

Instructions

1. Prepare the Mug: Spray a microwave safe mug with nonstick cooking spray.

2. Mix Ingredients: Add the egg whites, salmon, green onions, salt, and pepper to the mug. Stir to combine.

3. Microwave: Microwave on high for 12 minutes or until the eggs are set.

4. Serve: Enjoy directly from the mug or slide onto a plate.

Skinny Western Omelet Muffins

These Skinny Western Omelet Muffins are perfect for meal prep. Make a batch ahead of time for a quick, zeropoint breakfast that's ready to go whenever you are.

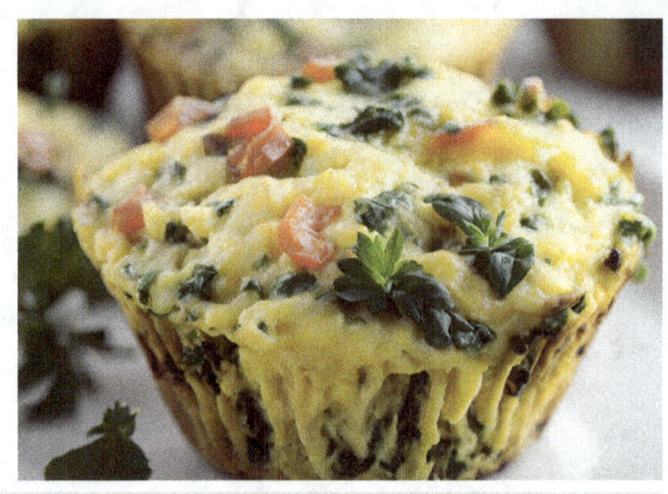

ingredients

- 1 cup egg whites
- 1/4 cup chopped bell peppers
- 1/4 cup chopped onions
- 1/4 cup diced ham (lean and lowfat)
- Salt and pepper to taste

Preparation Time
Total Time: 25 minutes

Cooking Time
20 minutes

Serving Size
6 muffins

Nutrition (per serving)
- Protein: 10g
- Carbs: 2g
- Fat: 1g

Instructions

1. Preheat Oven: Preheat your oven to 350°F (175°C).

2. Mix Ingredients: In a bowl, mix the egg whites, bell peppers, onions, ham, salt, and pepper.

3. Fill Muffin Tin: Pour the mixture into a nonstick muffin tin, filling each cup about three quarters full.

4. Bake: Bake for 1520 minutes or until the eggs are set.

5. Cool and Store: Let cool before storing in the refrigerator for up to 5 days.

Kodiak Cake Muffins

Kodiak Cake Muffins are a great way to enjoy a warm, satisfying breakfast packed with protein and flavor while still being low in calories and zero points

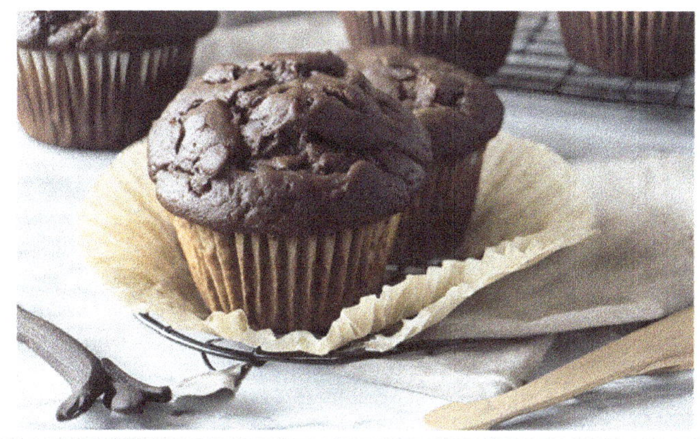

ingredients

- 1/2 cup Kodiak Cake mix
- 1/2 cup water
- 1/4 cup unsweetened applesauce
- 1 teaspoon baking powder

Preparation Time
Total Time: 25 minutes

Cooking Time
20 minutes

Serving Size
6 muffins

Nutrition (per serving)
- Protein: 7g
- Carbs: 12g
- Fat: 1g

Instructions

1. Preheat Oven: Preheat your oven to 350°F (175°C).

2. Mix Ingredients: In a bowl, combine the Kodiak Cake mix, water, applesauce, and baking powder. Stir until well combined.

3. Fill Muffin Tin: Pour the Batter into a nonstick muffin tin, filling each cup about three quarters full.

4. Bake: Bake for 1520 minutes or until a toothpick inserted into the center comes out clean.

5. Cool and Enjoy: Let cool before enjoying.

Cheesy Ham and Egg Cups

These Cheesy Ham and Egg Cups are a delightful, protein packed breakfast that's satisfying and easy to make. Perfect for busy mornings or meal prepping for the week.

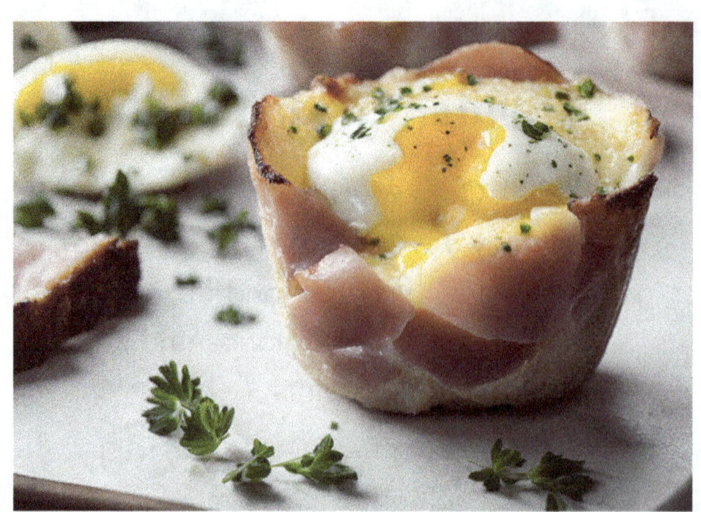

ingredients

- 6 slices lean ham
- 6 egg whites
- 1/4 cup shredded fat free cheese
- Salt and pepper to taste

Preparation Time

Total Time: 25 minutes

Cooking Time

20 minutes

Serving Size

6 cup

Nutrition (per serving)

- Protein: 10g
- Carbs: 1g
- Fat: 1g

Instructions

1. Preheat Oven: Preheat your oven to 350°F (175°C).

2. Line Muffin Tin: Line each cup of a nonstick muffin tin with a slice of ham.

3. Add Egg Whites: Pour egg whites into each ham cup, filling about threequarters full.

4. Top with Cheese: Sprinkle shredded cheese on each cup.

5. Bake: Bake for 1520 minutes or until the eggs are set.

6. Cool and Store: Let cool before storing in the refrigerator for up to 5 days.

W.W. Crepes

Indulge in these light and delicious W.W. Crepes. They're versatile and can be filled with your favorite fruits, making them a perfect zero point breakfast treat.

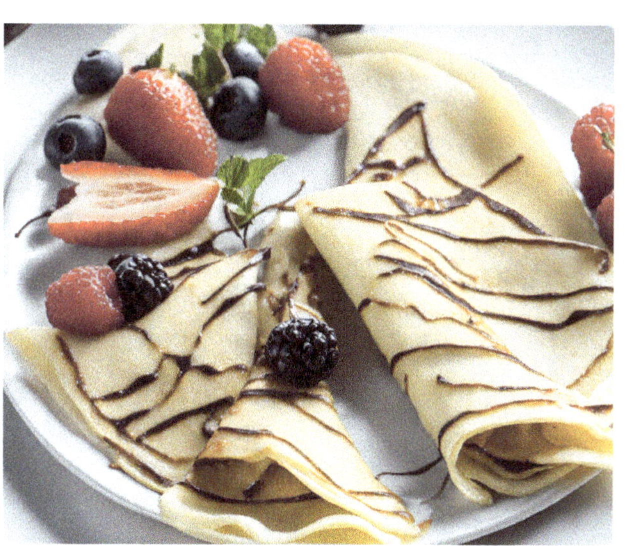

ingredients

- 1 cup egg whites
- 1/4 cup skim milk
- 1/2 cup all-purpose flour
- 1 teaspoon vanilla extract
- Cooking spray

Preparation Time
Total Time: 15 minutes

Cooking Time
10 minutes

Serving Size
4 crepes

Nutrition (per serving)

- Protein: 8g
- Carbs: 10g
- Fat: 0g

Instructions

1. Prepare Batter: In a bowl, whisk together egg whites, skim milk, flour, and vanilla extract until smooth.

2. Cook Crepes: Heat a nonstick skillet over medium heat and lightly coat with cooking spray. Pour a small amount of Batter into the skillet, tilting to spread evenly. Cook for 12 minutes until edges lift, then flip and cook for another 12 minutes.

3. Serve: Fill with fresh fruits and enjoy.

CHAPTER THREE

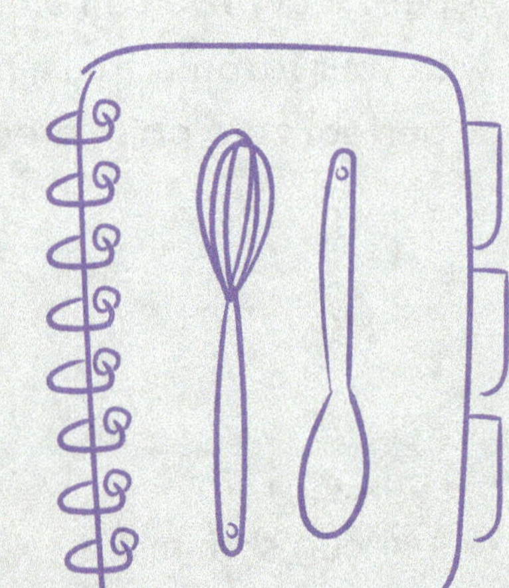

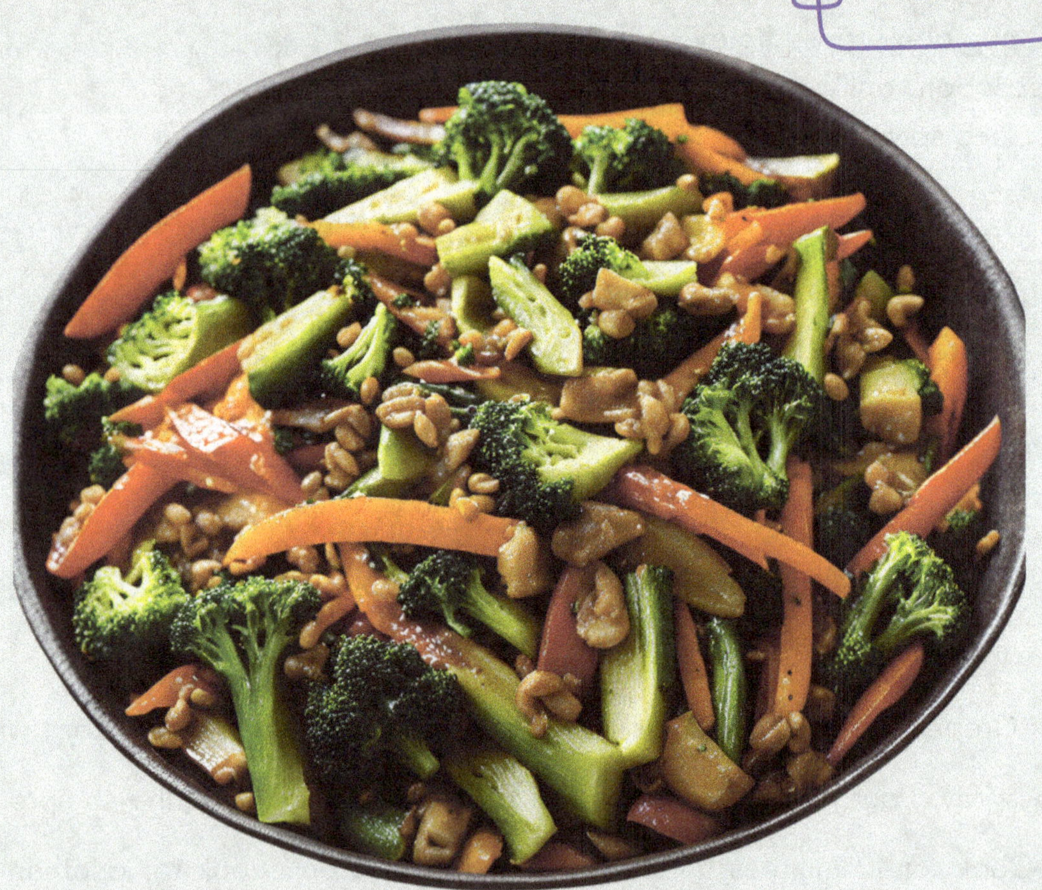

Lunch Recipes

Grilled Chicken Salad

Enjoy a hearty and refreshing Grilled Chicken Salad that's perfect for a light yet satisfying lunch. Packed with lean protein and crisp vegetables, this zero point meal will keep you full and energized throughout the day.

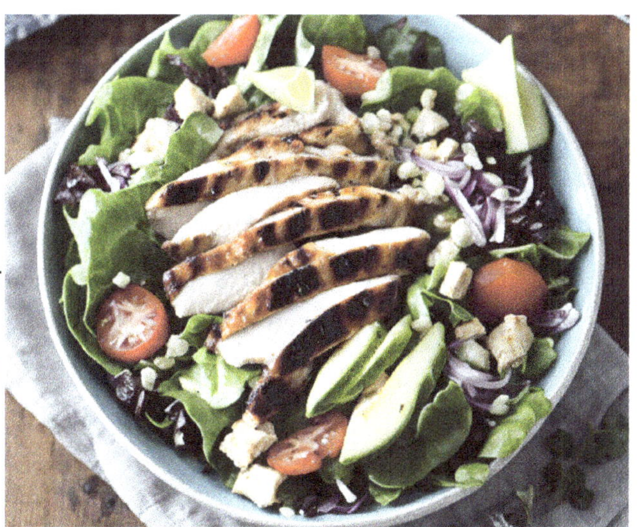

ingredients

- 1 skinless, boneless chicken breast
- 4 cups mixed greens (lettuce, Spinach, arugula)
- 1/2 cup cherry tomatoes, halved
- 1/4 cup sliced cucumbers
- 1/4 cup shredded carrots
- 1/4 cup sliced red onions
- 1 tablespoon balsamic vinegar
- Salt and pepper to taste

Preparation Time

Total Time: 15 minutes

Cooking Time

10 minutes

Serving Size

1

Nutrition (per serving)

- Protein: 30g
- Carbs: 10g
- Fat: 2g

Instructions

1. Grill the Chicken: Season the chicken breast with salt and pepper. Grill over medium high heat for 57 minutes on each side or until fully cooked. Let cool, then slice.

2. Prepare the Salad: In a large bowl, combine the mixed greens, cherry tomatoes, cucumbers, carrots, and red onions.

3. Assemble: Top the salad with the grilled chicken slices. Drizzle with balsamic vinegar and toss to combine.

4. Serve: Serve immediately and enjoy!

Vegetable StirFry

A quick and easy Vegetable Stir-fry is perfect for a nutritious and flavorful lunch. This zero point dish is packed with colorful veggies and can be made in under 15 minutes!

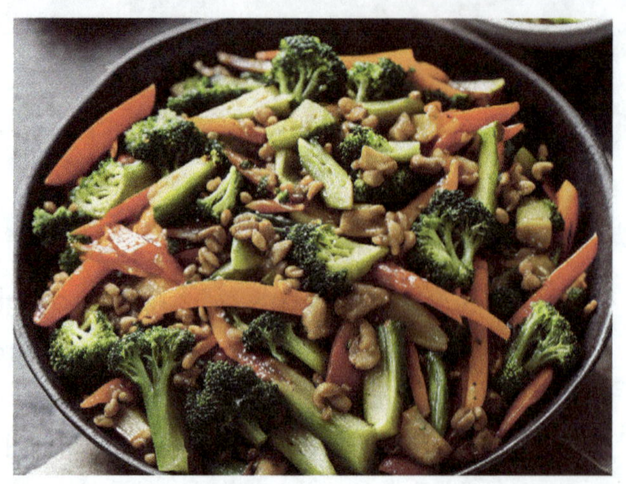

ingredients

- 1 cup broccoli florets
- 1/2 cup sliced bell peppers
- 1/2 cup sliced carrots
- 1/2 cup snap peas
- 1/4 cup sliced onions

- 2 cloves garlic, minced
- 1 tablespoon soy sauce
- 1 teaspoon sesame oil (optional)
- Salt and pepper to taste

Preparation Time
Total Time: 15 minutes

Cooking Time
10 minutes

Serving Size
2

Nutrition (per serving)
- Protein: 3g
- Carbs: 12g
- Fat: 2g

Instructions

1. Prepare Vegetables: Chop all the vegetables and set them aside.

2. Cook Vegetables: Heat the sesame oil over mediumhigh heat in a large nonstick skillet or wok. Add the garlic and onions, and sauté for 2 minutes.

3. Add Veggies: Add the broccoli, bell peppers, carrots, and snap peas. Stirfry for 57 minutes or until the vegetables are tendercrisp.

4. Season: Add soy sauce, salt, and pepper to taste. Stir well to combine.

5. Serve: Serve hot and enjoy!

Turkey Lettuce Wraps

Turkey Lettuce Wraps are a fun and delicious way to enjoy a low-calorie, high protein lunch. These wraps are fresh, crunchy, and flavorful, making them a zero-point favorite.

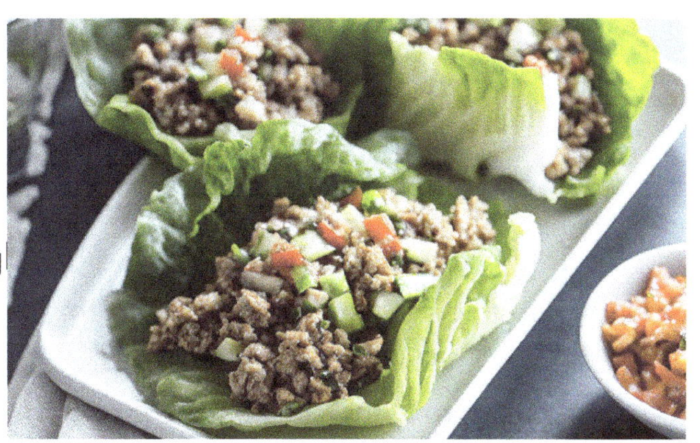

ingredients

- 1 cup cooked ground turkey breast
- 1/4 cup diced bell peppers
- 1/4 cup diced onions
- 1/4 cup shredded carrots
- 1 tablespoon soy sauce
- 1 teaspoon hoisin sauce
- 8 large lettuce leaves
- Salt and pepper to taste

Preparation Time

Total Time: 20 minutes

Cooking Time

15 minutes

Serving Size

2

Nutrition (per serving)

- Protein: 20g
- Carbs: 5g
- Fat: 2g

Instructions

1. Prepare Filling: In a nonstick skillet, cook the ground turkey, bell peppers, onions, and carrots over medium heat until the turkey is fully cooked, about 710 minutes.

2. Season: Add the soy sauce, hoisin sauce, salt, and pepper. Stir to combine and cook for another 2 minutes.

3. Assemble Wraps: Spoon the turkey mixture into the center of each lettuce leaf.

4. Serve: Roll up the lettuce leaves and enjoy immediately.

Quinoa and Black Bean Salad

This Quinoa and Black Bean Salad is a refreshing and satisfying zero point lunch. The combination of protein packed quinoa and fiber rich black beans makes it a perfect meal to keep you going all day.

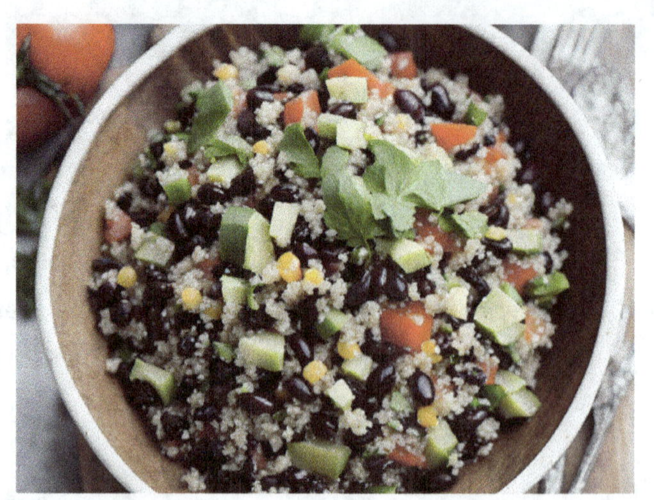

ingredients

- 1 cup cooked quinoa
- 1 cup canned black beans, rinsed and drained
- 1/2 cup corn kernels
- 1/4 cup diced red bell pepper
- 1/4 cup chopped cilantro
- 1/4 cup diced red onion
- Juice of 1 lime
- Salt and pepper to taste

Preparation Time
Total Time: 20 minutes

Cooking Time
15 minutes

Serving Size
2

Nutrition (per serving)
- Protein: 8g
- Carbs: 28g
- Fat: 2g

Instructions

1. Prepare Ingredients: Cook the quinoa according to package instructions and let cool.

2. Mix Salad: In a large bowl, combine the cooked quinoa, black beans, corn, bell pepper, cilantro, and red onion.

3. Season: Add lime juice, salt, and pepper. Toss to combine.

4. Serve: Serve immediately or chill in the refrigerator before serving.

Cucumber and Tomato Salad

Light and refreshing, this Cucumber and Tomato Salad is a perfect zero point lunch. Its crisp textures and vibrant flavors make it a delightful way to enjoy your vegetables.

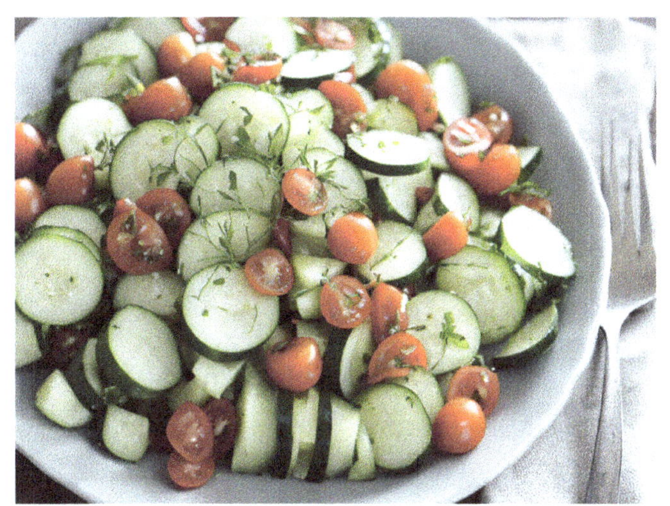

ingredients

- 1 cucumber, sliced
- 1 cup cherry tomatoes, halved
- 1/4 cup sliced red onion
- 2 tablespoons chopped fresh dill
- 1 tablespoon red wine vinegar
- Salt and pepper to taste

Preparation Time

Total Time: 10 minutes

Cooking Time

None

Serving Size

2

Nutrition (per serving)

- Protein: 1g
- Carbs: 8g
- Fat: 0g

Instructions

1. Prepare Vegetables: Slice the cucumber, halve the cherry tomatoes, and slice the red onion.

2. Mix Salad: In a large bowl, combine the cucumber, cherry tomatoes, red onion, and dill.

3. Season: Add red wine vinegar, salt, and pepper. Toss to combine.

4. Serve: Serve immediately.

Chipotle Chicken Casserole

Spice up your lunch with this flavorful Chipotle Chicken Casserole. It's a hearty and delicious zero point meal that will satisfy your taste buds.

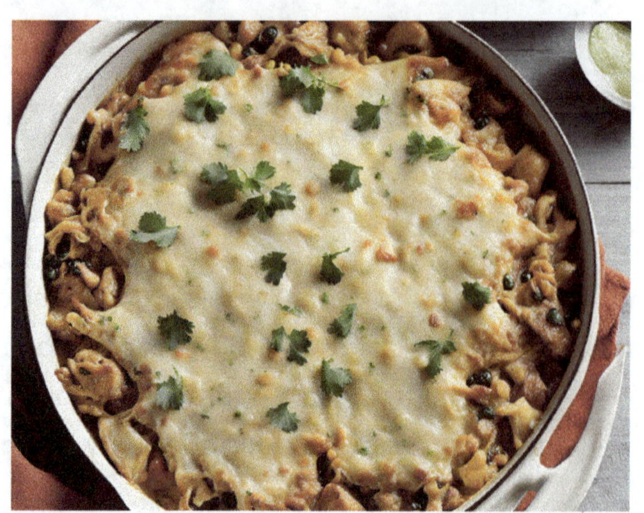

ingredients

- 2 skinless, boneless chicken breasts, cooked and shredded
- 1 can diced tomatoes with green chilies
- 1/2 cup black beans, rinsed and drained
- 1/2 cup corn kernels
- 1/4 cup diced red onion
- 1 teaspoon chipotle powder
- 1/2 teaspoon cumin
- Salt and pepper to taste

Preparation Time

Total Time: 30 minutes

Cooking Time

20 minutes

Serving Size

2

Nutrition (per serving)

- Protein: 1g
- Carbs: 8g
- Fat: 0g

Instructions

1. Preheat Oven: Preheat your oven to 350°F (175°C).

2. Mix Ingredients: In a large bowl, combine the shredded Chicken, diced tomatoes, black beans, corn, red onion, chipotle powder, cumin, salt, and pepper.

3. Bake: Transfer the mixture to a baking dish and bake for 20 minutes or until heated.

4. Serve: Serve hot and enjoy!

Grilled Crab Legs

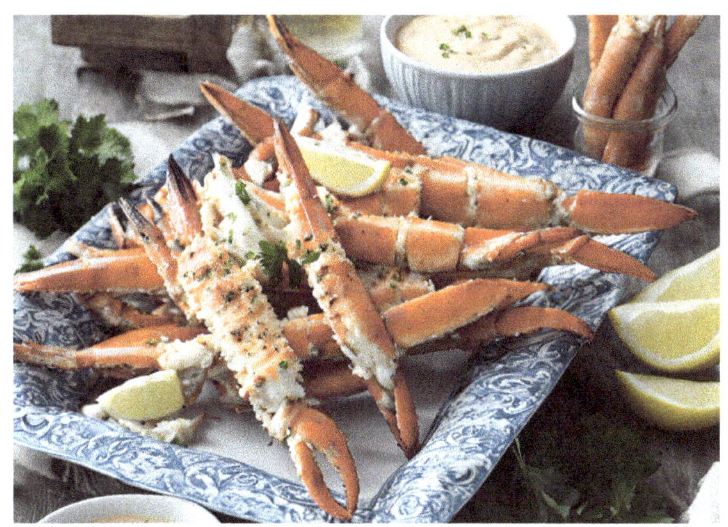

Indulge in a luxurious and light lunch with these Grilled Crab Legs. They're simple to prepare, rich in flavor, and make a perfect meal.

ingredients

- 4 crab legs
- 1 lemon, cut into wedges
- 1 tablespoon fresh parsley, chopped
- Salt and pepper to taste

Preparation Time

Total Time: 15 minutes

Cooking Time

10 minutes

Serving Size

2

Nutrition (per serving)

- Protein: 22g
- Carbs: 2g
- Fat: 2g

Instructions

1. Preheat Grill: Preheat your Grill to medium high heat.

2. Grill Crab Legs: Place the crab legs on the Grill and cook for 57 minutes on each side or until heated.

3. Season: Remove from the Grill and sprinkle with fresh parsley, salt, and pepper.

4. Serve: Serve with lemon wedges

Baked Zucchini Chips

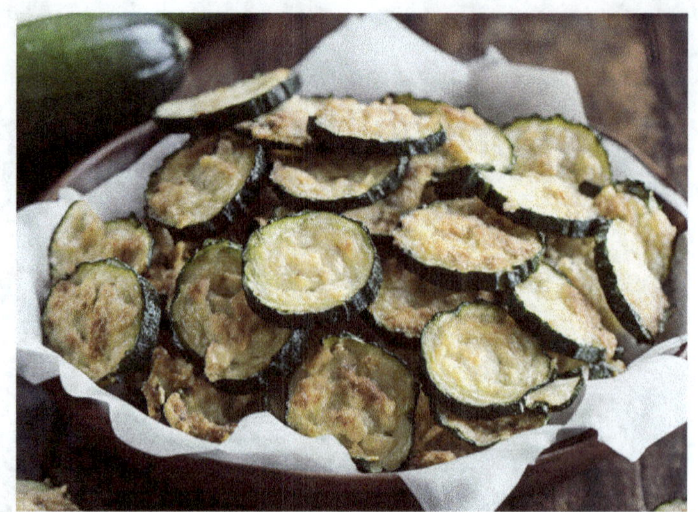

Satisfy your crunchy cravings with these Baked Zucchini Chips. They are a perfect low-calorie, snack or side dish that's easy to make and deliciously addictive.

ingredients

- 2 medium zucchinis
- 1 teaspoon garlic powder
- 1 teaspoon paprika
- Salt and pepper to taste

Preparation Time

Total Time: 2 hours 10 minutes

Cooking Time

2 hours

Serving Size

4

Nutrition (per serving)

- Protein: 1g
- Carbs: 4g
- Fat: 0g

Instructions

1. Preheat Oven: Preheat your oven to 225°F (110°C).

2. Prepare Zucchini: Slice the Zucchini into thin rounds.

3. Season: Place the zucchini slices in a bowl and toss with garlic powder, paprika, salt, and pepper.

4. Bake: Arrange the zucchini slices on a baking sheet lined with parchment paper. Bake for 1.5 to 2 hours or until crispy.

5. Cool and Serve: Let cool before serving.

Jello Grapes

This Jello Grapes recipe turns your ordinary grapes into a fun, colorful snack. It's a sweet and tangy treat that is perfect for satisfying your cravings without guilt.

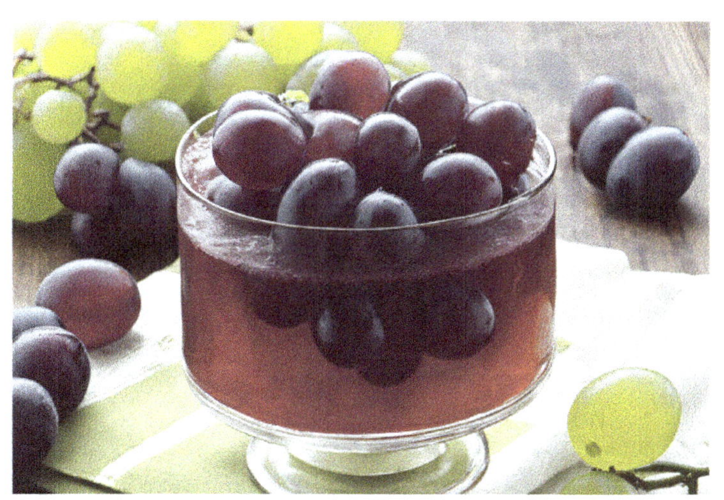

ingredients

- 2 cups green or red grapes, washed and dried
- 1 package sugar free Jello powder (any flavor)

Preparation Time

Total Time: 1 hour 5 minutes

Cooking Time

None

Serving Size

4

Nutrition (per serving)

- Protein: 0g
- Carbs: 10g
- Fat: 0g

Instructions

1. Prepare Grapes: Wash and thoroughly dry the grapes.

2. Coat with Jell: Place the grapes in a large ziplock bag and add the Jello powder. Shake well to coat the grapes evenly.

3. Chill: Spread the coated grapes on a baking sheet and refrigerate for at least 1 hour.

4. Serve: Enjoy these chilled, sweet treats.

Lemon Greek Chicken Skewers

Infuse your lunch with Mediterranean flavors with these Lemon Greek Chicken Skewers. Marinated in a tangy lemon herb mixture, they're delicious, healthy, and zero points.

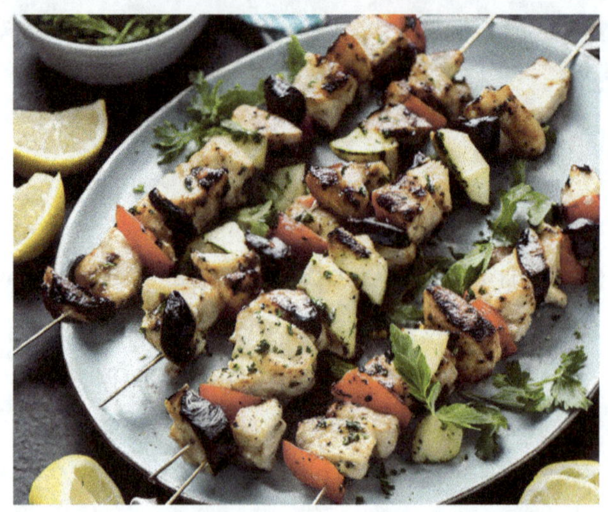

ingredients

- 2 skinless, boneless chicken breasts cut into cubes
- Juice of 1 lemon
- 2 cloves garlic, minced
- 1 teaspoon dried oregano
- Salt and pepper to taste
- Wooden skewers soaked in water

Preparation Time

45 minutes

Cooking Time

12 minutes

Serving Size

2

Nutrition (per serving)

- Protein: 24g
- Carbs: 2g
- Fat: 3g

Instructions

1. Marinate Chicken: In a bowl, mix lemon juice, garlic, oregano, salt, and pepper. Add chicken cubes and marinate for at least 30 minutes.

2. Prepare Skewers: Thread the marinated Chicken onto the soaked skewers.

3. Grill Skewers: Preheat the Grill to medium high heat and grill the skewers for about 1012 minutes, turning occasionally, until the Chicken is cooked through.

4. Serve: Serve immediately with a side salad or veggies.

Egg Salad

A classic Egg Salad made healthier! This zero point version uses Greek yogurt instead of mayo, making it a perfect quick and nutritious lunch option.

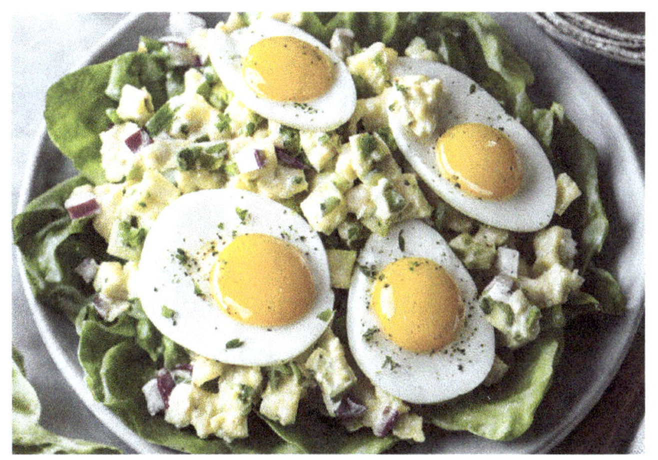

ingredients

- 4 hardboiled eggs, chopped
- 1/4 cup fat free Greek yogurt
- 1 tablespoon Dijon mustard
- 1 tablespoon chopped fresh chives
- Salt and pepper to taste

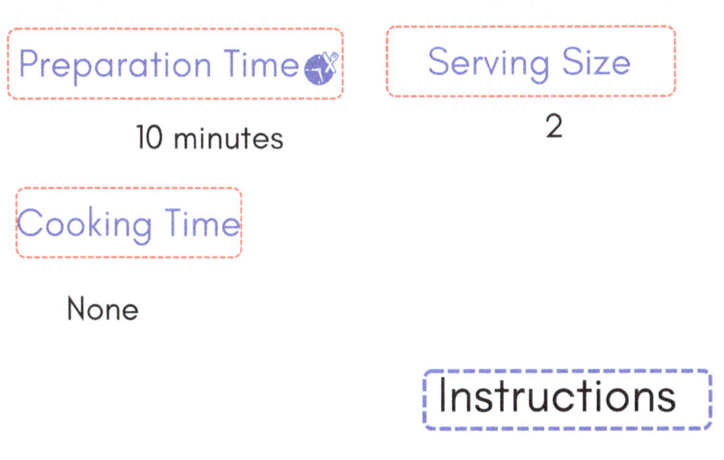

Preparation Time

10 minutes

Cooking Time

None

Serving Size

2

Nutrition (per serving)

- Protein: 12g
- Carbs: 2g
- Fat: 2g

Instructions

1. Prepare Eggs: Chop the hardboiled eggs and place them in a bowl.

2. Mix Ingredients: Add Greek yogurt, Dijon mustard, chives, salt, and pepper to the eggs. Mix well until combined.

3. Serve: Serve immediately or chill in the refrigerator before serving.

One Pan Chicken Fajitas

Enjoy the bold flavors of fajitas without the fuss with this Pan Chicken Fajitas recipe. It's a quick, easy, perfect for lunch or dinner

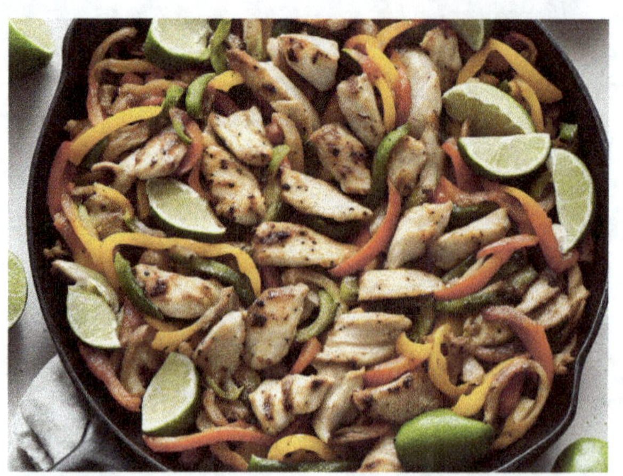

ingredients

- 2 skinless, boneless chicken breasts, sliced
- 1 red bell pepper, sliced
- 1 green bell pepper, sliced
- 1 yellow bell pepper, sliced
- 1 onion, sliced
- 2 cloves garlic, minced
- 1 tablespoon chili powder
- 1 teaspoon cumin
- 1 teaspoon paprika
- Salt and pepper to taste

Preparation Time

30 minutes

Cooking Time

25 minutes

Serving Size

4

Nutrition (per serving)

- Protein: 25g
- Carbs: 8g
- Fat: 2g

Instructions

1. Preheat Oven: Preheat your oven to 400°F (200°C).

2. Mix Ingredients: In a large bowl, combine the Chicken, bell peppers, onion, garlic, chili powder, cumin, paprika, salt, and pepper. Toss until well coated.

3. Bake: Spread the mixture on a baking sheet and bake for 2025 minutes, or until the Chicken is cooked and the vegetables are tender.

4. Serve: Serve with lettuce wraps or over a bed of greens.

3 Bean Turkey Chili

Warm up with a hearty bowl of 3Bean Turkey Chili. This zero point recipe is rich in flavor and packed with protein and fiber, making it a perfect lunch option

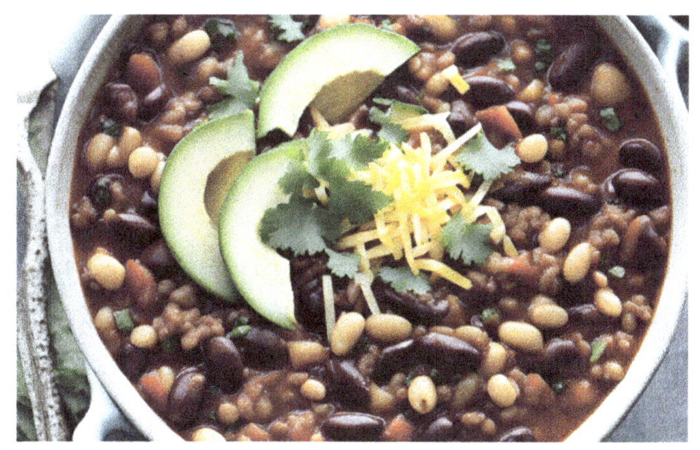

ingredients

- 1 pound ground turkey breast
- 1 can black beans, rinsed and drained
- 1 can kidney beans, rinsed and drained
- 1 can pinto beans, rinsed and drained
- 1 can diced tomatoes
- 1 onion, diced
- 2 cloves garlic, minced
- 1 tablespoon chili powder
- 1 teaspoon cumin
- Salt and pepper to taste

Preparation Time
35 minutes

Cooking Time
20 minutes

Serving Size
4

Nutrition (per serving)
- Protein: 25g
- Carbs: 8g
- Fat: 2g

Instructions

1. Cook Turkey: In a large pot, cook the ground turkey over medium heat until browned.

2. Add Ingredients: Add the onion and garlic, and cook until softened, about 5 minutes.

3. Combine Beans and Spices: Add the black beans, kidney beans, pinto beans, diced tomatoes, chili powder, cumin, salt, and pepper. Stir to combine.

4. Simmer: Bring to a boil, then reduce heat and simmer for 20 minutes.

5. Serve: Serve hot, garnished with fresh cilantro or green onions if desired.   38

Chicken Enchilada Stuffed Zucchini

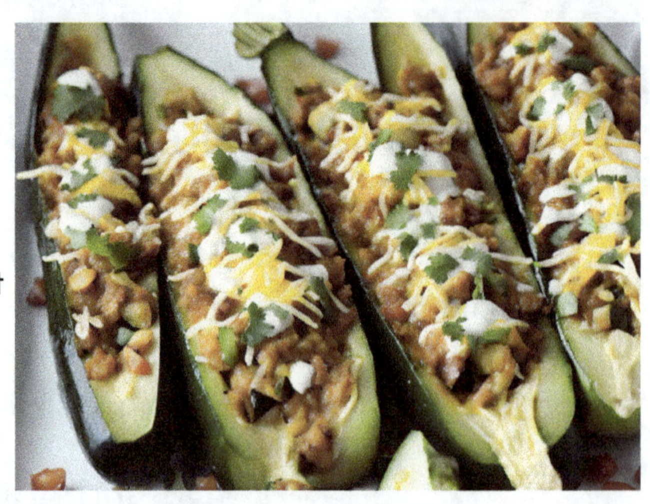

Enjoy the flavors of enchiladas without the carbs with these Chicken enchiladas stuffed with Zucchini. They're a delightful lunch option that's both healthy and tasty.

ingredients

- 2 medium zucchinis, halved lengthwise and seeds scooped out
- 1 cup cooked, shredded chicken breast
- 1/2 cup enchilada sauce
- 1/4 cup diced tomatoes
- 1/4 cup black beans, rinsed and drained
- 1/4 cup corn kernels
- 1/4 cup shredded fatfree cheese (optional)
- Fresh cilantro for garnish

Preparation Time

30 minutes

Cooking Time

20 minutes

Serving Size

2

Nutrition (per serving)

- Protein: 22g
- Carbs: 15g
- Fat: 2g

Instructions

1. Preheat Oven: Preheat your oven to 375°F (190°C).

2. Prepare Zucchini: Scoop out the seeds of the zucchini halves to create boats.

3. Mix Filling: In a bowl, combine the shredded Chicken, enchilada sauce, diced tomatoes, black beans, and corn.

4. Stuff Zucchini: Fill each zucchini half with the chicken mixture and place on a baking sheet.

5. Bake: Bake for 20 minutes. If using cheese, sprinkle on top during the last 5 minutes of baking.

6. Serve: Garnish with fresh cilantro and serve hot.

Buffalo Chicken Lettuce Wraps

Buffalo Chicken Lettuce Wraps are a spicy and crunchy zeropoint lunch that's quick to make and flavorful. Perfect for those who love a bit of heat in their meals.

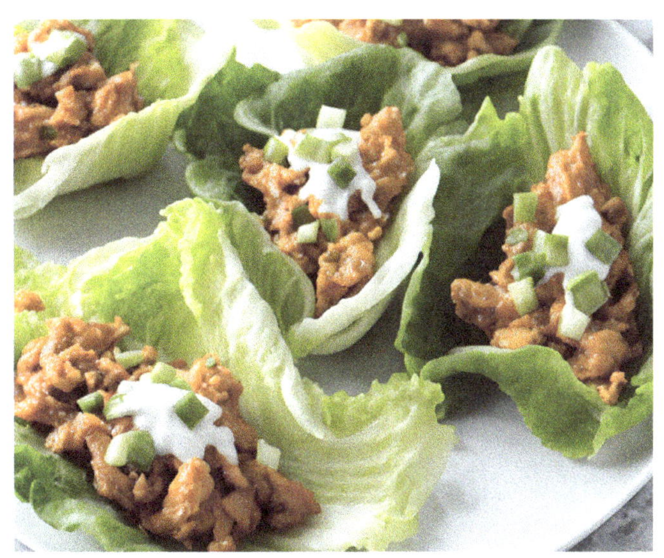

ingredients

- 2 cups cooked, shredded chicken breast
- 1/4 cup hot sauce (such as Frank's RedHot)
- 1/4 cup fatfree Greek yogurt
- 8 large lettuce leaves
- 1/4 cup diced celery
- 1/4 cup diced carrots
- 1 tablespoon ranch seasoning mix

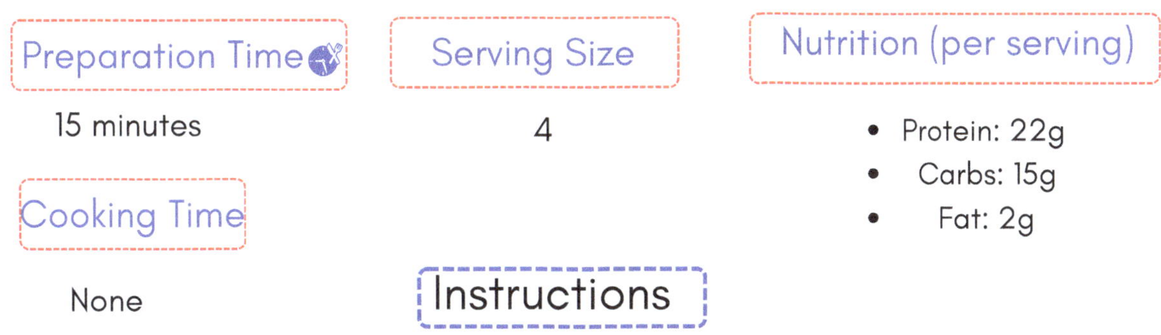

Preparation Time
15 minutes

Cooking Time
None

Serving Size
4

Nutrition (per serving)
- Protein: 22g
- Carbs: 15g
- Fat: 2g

Instructions

1. Prepare Chicken: In a bowl, mix the shredded Chicken with hot sauce, Greek yogurt, and ranch seasoning until well combined.

2. Assemble Wraps: Place a spoonful of the buffalo chicken mixture onto each lettuce leaf.

3. Add Veggies: Top with diced celery and carrots.

4. Serve: Wrap the lettuce around the filling and enjoy immediately.

CHAPTER FOUR

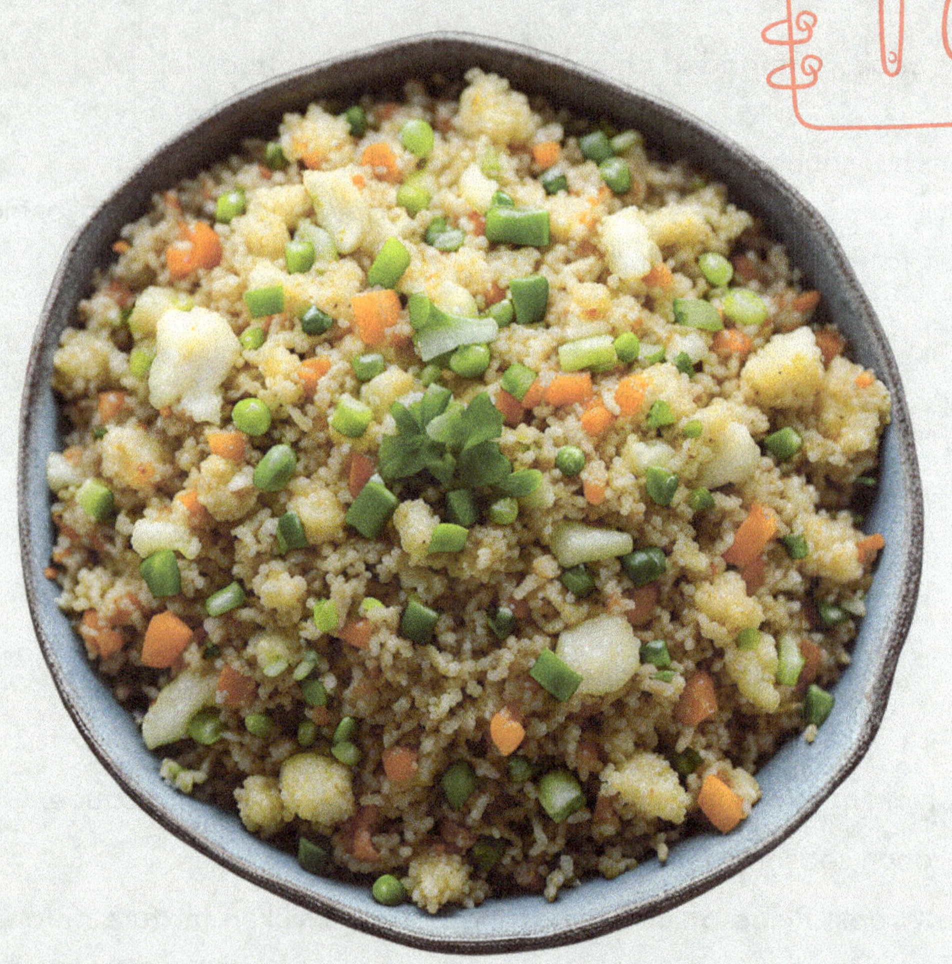

Dinner Recipes

Baked Salmon with Asparagus

Enjoy a delicious and nutritious dinner with this Baked Salmon with Asparagus recipe. It's a zero point meal packed with flavor and essential nutrients, making it a perfect choice for a healthy lifestyle.

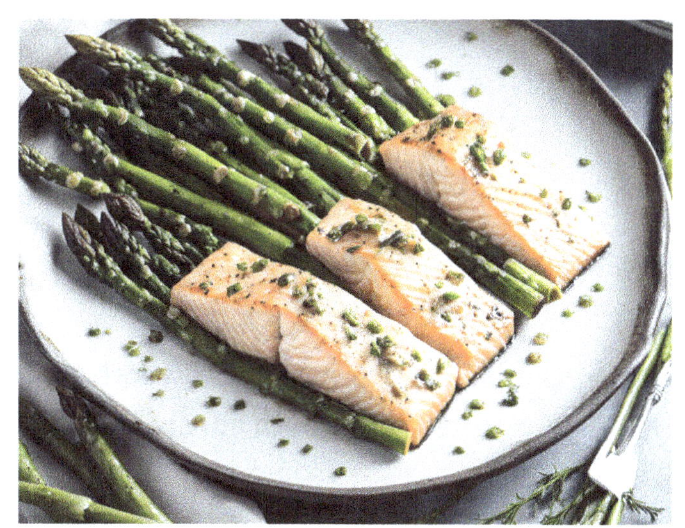

ingredients

- 2 salmon fillets
- 1 bunch asparagus, trimmed
- 2 cloves garlic, minced
- Juice of 1 lemon
- 1 teaspoon dried dill
- Salt and pepper to taste

Preparation Time

25 minutes

Cooking Time

20 minutes

Serving Size

2

Nutrition (per serving)

- Protein: 30g
- Carbs: 5g
- Fat: 10g

Instructions

1. Preheat Oven: Preheat your oven to 400°F (200°C).

2. Prepare Baking Sheet: Line a baking sheet with parchment paper. Arrange the salmon fillets and asparagus on the sheet.

3. Season: Drizzle the lemon juice over the salmon and asparagus. Sprinkle with garlic, dill, salt, and pepper.

4. Bake: Bake for 1520 minutes until the salmon is cooked and the asparagus is tender.

5. Serve: Serve immediately, garnished with additional lemon slices if desired.

Zucchini Noodles with Marinara Sauce

Replace traditional pasta with these healthy Zucchini Noodles with Marinara Sauce. It's a zero point, lowcarb dinner option that's both satisfying and delicious.

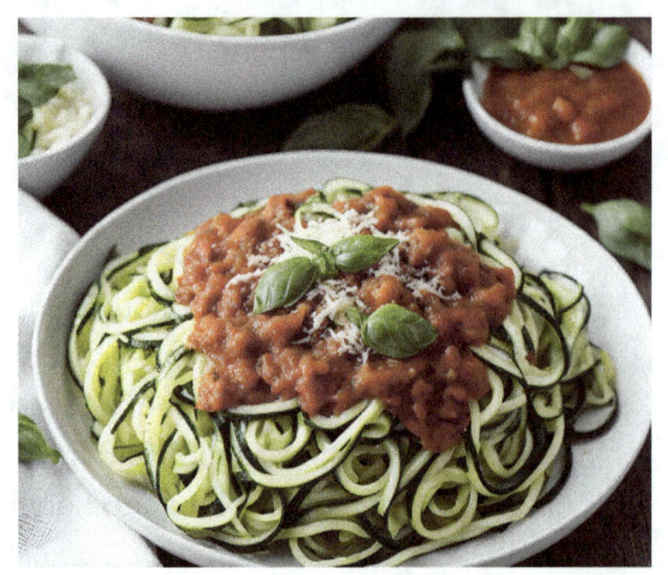

ingredients

- 2 large zucchinis, spiralized
- 2 cups marinara sauce (sugarfree)
- 1/4 cup chopped fresh basil
- 1/4 cup grated Parmesan cheese (optional)
- Salt and pepper to taste
-

Preparation Time

15 minutes

Cooking Time

3 minutes

Serving Size

2

Nutrition (per serving)

- Protein: 4g
- Carbs: 14g
- Fat: 2g

Instructions

1. Prepare Zucchini Noodles: Spiralize the zucchinis to create noodles. Set aside.

2. Heat Marinara Sauce: In a large skillet, heat the marinara sauce over medium heat until simmering.

3. Cook Zoodles: Add the zucchini noodles to the skillet and toss to coat in the sauce. Cook for 23 minutes until tender.

4. Serve: Serve immediately, topped with fresh basil and Parmesan cheese if desired.

Chicken and Vegetable Skewers

Enjoy a flavorful and healthy dinner with these Chicken and Vegetable Skewers. This recipe is perfect for grilling season and can be easily customized with your favorite veggies.

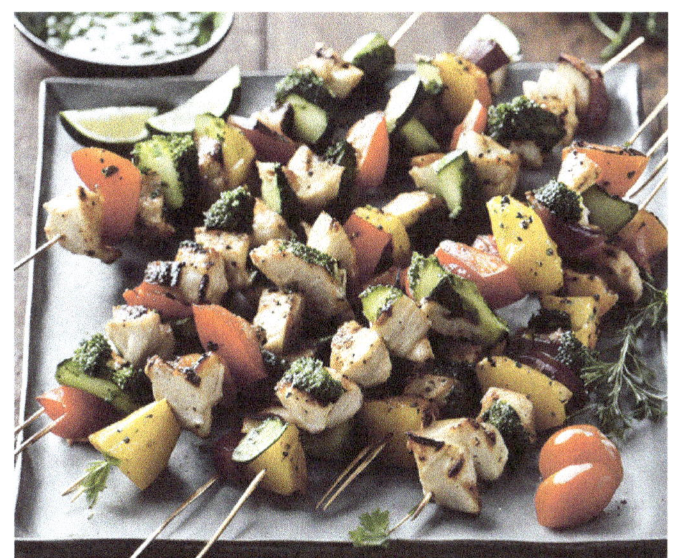

ingredients

- 2 skinless, boneless chicken breasts cut into cubes
- 1 red bell pepper, cut into chunks
- 1 yellow bell pepper, cut into chunks
- 1 zucchini, sliced
- 1 red onion, cut into chunks
- 1/4 cup olive oil
- Juice of 1 lemon
- 2 cloves garlic, minced
- 1 teaspoon dried oregano
- Salt and pepper to taste
- Wooden skewers soaked in water

Preparation Time

45 minutes

Cooking Time

12 minutes

Serving Size

4

Nutrition (per serving)

- Protein: 20g
- Carbs: 5g
- Fat: 5g

Instructions

1. Marinate Chicken: In a bowl, combine olive oil, lemon juice, garlic, oregano, salt, and pepper. Add Chicken and vegetables, tossing to coat. Marinate for at least 30 minutes.

2. Prepare Skewers: Thread the marinated Chicken and vegetables onto the soaked skewers.

3. Grill Skewers: Preheat grill to medium high heat. Grill the skewers for 1012 minutes, turning occasionally, until the Chicken is cooked and the vegetables are tender.

4. Serve: Serve immediately with a salad or rice.

Stuffed Bell Peppers

These Stuffed Bell Peppers are a hearty and nutritious dinner option. Filled with a savory mixture of ground turkey and vegetables, they're a zero point meal sure to satisfy.

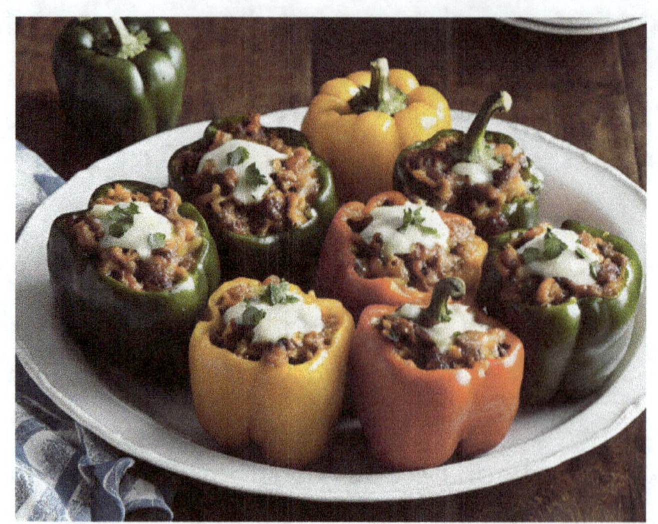

ingredients

- 4 bell peppers, tops cut off and seeds removed
- 1 pound ground turkey breast
- 1 onion, diced
- 1 cup cooked quinoa
- 1 teaspoon cumin
- 1 teaspoon chili powder
- Salt and pepper to taste
- Fresh cilantro for garnish
- 1 can diced tomatoes

Preparation Time

40 minutes

Cooking Time

30 minutes

Serving Size

4

Nutrition (per serving)

- Protein: 25g
- Carbs: 20g
- Fat: 2g

Instructions

1. Preheat Oven: Preheat your oven to 375°F (190°C).

2. Cook Turkey: In a large skillet, cook the ground turkey and onion over medium heat until browned.

3. Mix Filling: Add the cooked quinoa, diced tomatoes, cumin, chili powder, salt, and pepper to the skillet. Stir to combine.

4. Stuff Peppers: Fill each bell pepper with the turkey mixture and place in a baking dish.

5. Bake: Bake for 2530 minutes or until the peppers are tender.

6. Serve: Garnish with fresh cilantro and serve hot.

Cauliflower Fried Rice

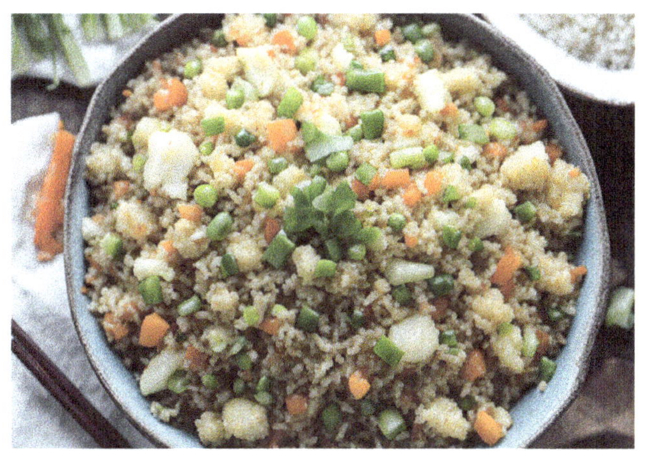

Enjoy a lowcarb version of a classic favorite with this Cauliflower Fried Rice. It's a quick and easy zeropoint dinner packed with vegetables and flavor.

ingredients

- 1 head cauliflower, grated into rice sized pieces
- 1 cup frozen peas and carrots
- 1/2 cup chopped onions
- 2 cloves garlic, minced
- 2 eggs, beaten
- 2 tablespoons soy sauce
- 1 teaspoon sesame oil
- Salt and pepper to taste
- Green onions for garnish

Preparation Time

20 minutes

Cooking Time

10 minutes

Serving Size

4

Nutrition (per serving)

- Protein: 6g
- Carbs: 12g
- Fat: 3g

Instructions

1. Prepare Cauliflower Rice: Grate the cauliflower into ricesized pieces and set aside.

2. Cook Vegetables: Heat the sesame oil over mediumhigh heat in a large skillet or wok. Add the onions and garlic, and cook for 23 minutes until fragrant.

3. Add Cauliflower Rice: Add the grated cauliflower, frozen peas, and carrots. Cook for 57 minutes, stirring frequently, until the vegetables are tender.

4. Scramble Eggs: Push the cauliflower mixture to the side of the skillet and pour the beaten eggs into the space. Scramble the eggs until cooked, then mix them into the cauliflower rice.

5. Season: Add soy sauce, salt, and pepper, and stir well to combine.

6. Serve: Garnish with green onions and serve hot.

Slow Cooker Tomato Balsamic Chicken

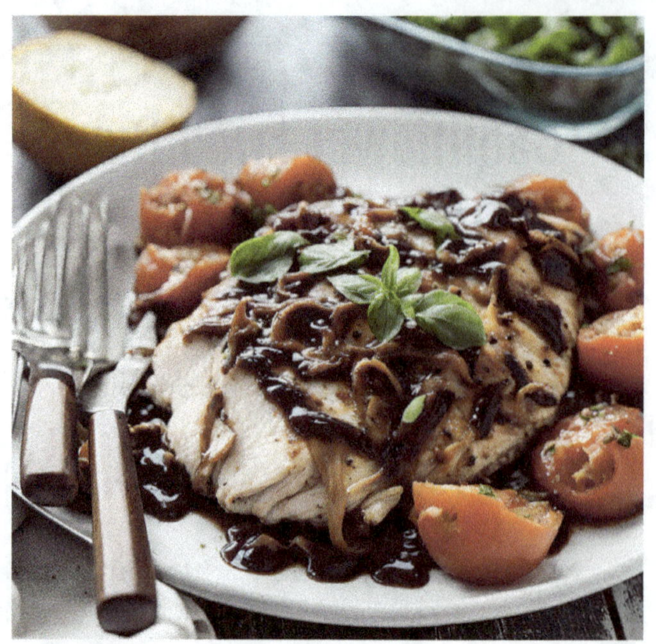

This Slow Cooker Tomato Balsamic Chicken is a savory and tangy dish perfect for a hassle-free dinner. Set it in the morning and return to a delicious meal.

ingredients

- 2 skinless, boneless chicken breasts
- 1 can diced tomatoes
- 1/4 cup balsamic vinegar
- 1 onion, diced

- 2 cloves garlic, minced
- 1 teaspoon dried basil
- 1 teaspoon dried oregano
- Salt and pepper to taste

Preparation Time

68 hours

Cooking Time

68 hours

Serving Size

4

Nutrition (per serving)

- Protein: 30g
- Carbs: 10g
- Fat: 4g

Instructions

1. Prepare Ingredients: Place the chicken breasts in the slow cooker.

2. Add Vegetables and Seasonings: Add the diced tomatoes, balsamic vinegar, onion, garlic, basil, oregano, salt, and pepper.

3. Cook: Cover and cook on low for 68 hours or on high for 34 hours.

4. Serve: Serve hot over a bed of steamed vegetables or rice.

Turkey, Corn, and Black Bean Chili

Warm up with this hearty Turkey, Corn, and Black Bean Chili. It's a protein packed, dinner full of flavor and perfect for a cozy night.

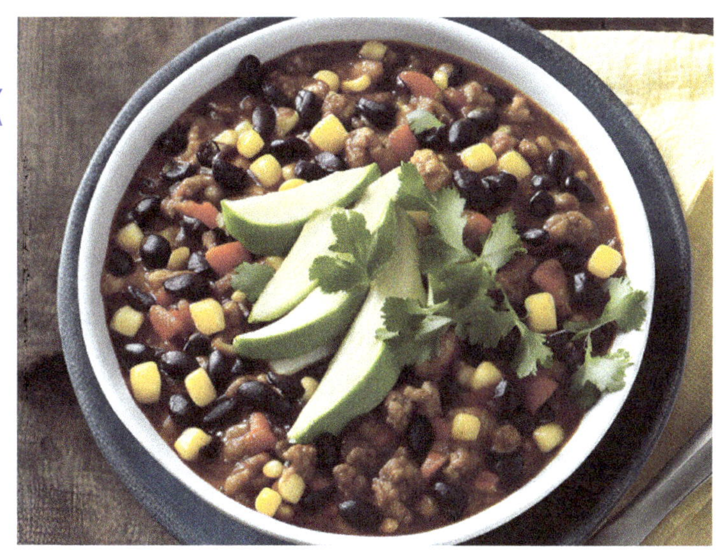

ingredients

- 1 pound ground turkey breast
- 1 can black beans, rinsed and drained
- 1 can corn, drained
- 1 can diced tomatoes
- 1 onion, diced
- 2 cloves garlic, minced
- 1 tablespoon chili powder
- 1 teaspoon cumin
- Salt and pepper to taste

Preparation Time

30 minutes

Cooking Time

20 minutes

Serving Size

4

Nutrition (per serving)

- Protein: 30g
- Carbs: 10g
- Fat: 4g

Instructions

1. Cook Turkey: In a large pot, cook the ground turkey over medium heat until browned.

2. Add Ingredients: Add the onion, garlic, black beans, corn, diced tomatoes, chili powder, cumin, salt, and pepper.

3. Simmer: Bring to a boil, then reduce heat and simmer for 20 minutes.

4. Serve: Serve hot, garnished with fresh cilantro or cheese if desired.

Lentil Soup

This hearty Lentil Soup is a warming, nutritious, dinner perfect for a chilly evening. It's easy to make and packed with protein and fiber.

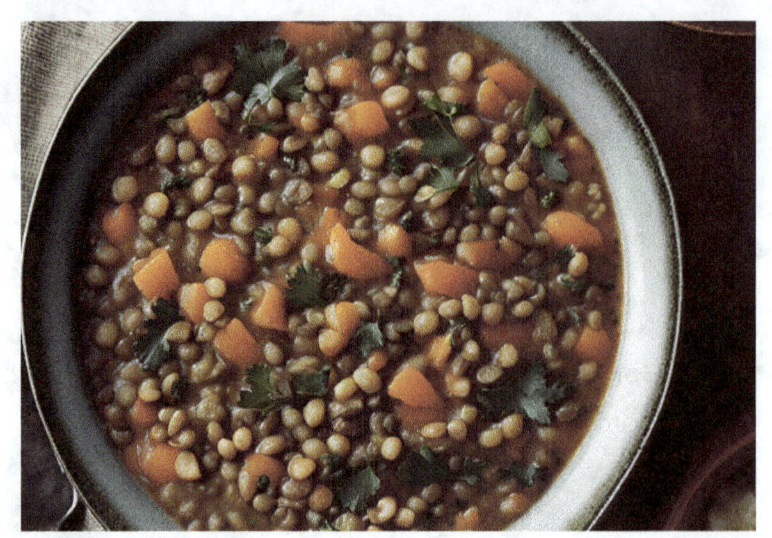

ingredients

- 1 cup lentils, rinsed
- 1 carrot, diced
- 1 celery stalk, diced
- 1 onion, diced
- 2 cloves garlic, minced
- 1 can diced tomatoes
- 4 cups vegetable broth
- 1 teaspoon cumin
- 1 teaspoon thyme
- Salt and pepper to taste

Preparation Time

45 minutes

Cooking Time

40 minutes

Serving Size

4

Nutrition (per serving)

- Protein: 12g
- Carbs: 30g
- Fat: 2g

Instructions

1. Prepare Vegetables: In a large pot, sauté the onion, carrot, celery, and garlic until softened.

2. Add Ingredients: Add the lentils, diced tomatoes, vegetable broth, cumin, thyme, salt, and pepper.

3. Simmer: Bring to a boil, then reduce heat and simmer for 3040 minutes, or until the lentils are tender.

4. Serve: Serve hot, garnished with fresh parsley if desired.

Garden Vegetable Soup

This Garden Vegetable Soup is a delightful way to enjoy a variety of fresh vegetables. It's a zero point, nutrient rich dinner that's light yet satisfying.

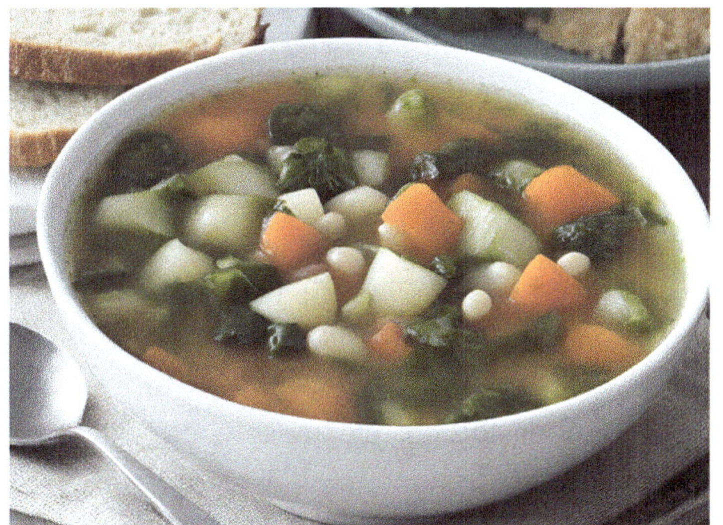

ingredients

- 1 cup diced carrots
- 1 cup diced celery
- 1 cup diced zucchini
- 1 cup diced tomatoes
- 1 cup green beans, cut into pieces
- 1 onion, diced

- 2 cloves garlic, minced
- 4 cups vegetable broth
- 1 teaspoon thyme
- Salt and pepper to taste

Preparation Time

30 minutes

Cooking Time

25 minutes

Serving Size

4

Nutrition (per serving)

- Protein: 3g
- Carbs: 20g
- Fat: 1g

Instructions

1. Prepare Vegetables: In a large pot, sauté the onion, carrots, celery, and garlic until softened.

2. Add Ingredients: Add the zucchini, tomatoes, green beans, vegetable broth, thyme, salt, and pepper.

3. Simmer: Bring to a boil, then reduce heat and simmer for 2025 minutes or until the vegetables are tender.

4. Serve: Serve hot, garnished with fresh basil if desired.

Crockpot Bean Soup

This Crockpot Bean Soup is a simple, delicious dinner you can set and forget. It's packed with fiber and protein, making it a satisfying and healthy meal.

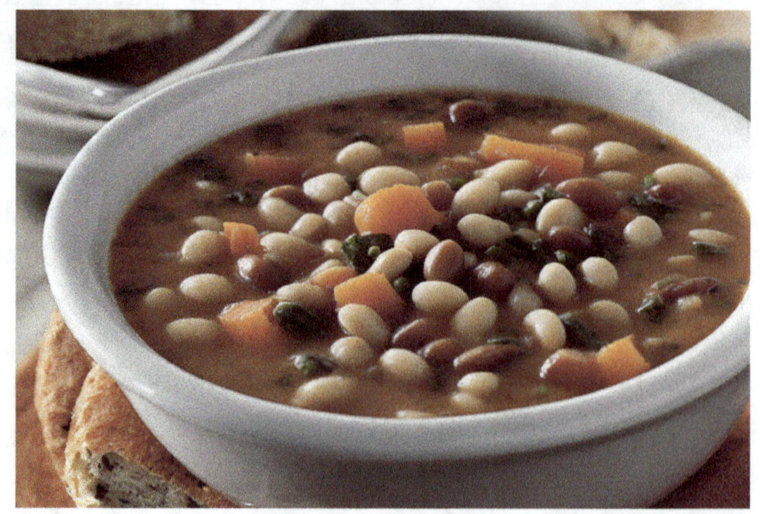

ingredients

- 1 can black beans, rinsed and drained
- 1 can kidney beans, rinsed and drained
- 1 can pinto beans, rinsed and drained
- 1 can diced tomatoes
- 1 onion, diced
- 2 cloves garlic, minced
- 4 cups vegetable broth
- 1 teaspoon cumin
- 1 teaspoon oregano
- Salt and pepper to taste

Preparation Time

68 hours

Cooking Time

68 hours

Serving Size

4

Nutrition (per serving)

- Protein: 10g
- Carbs: 30g
- Fat: 1g

Instructions

1. Prepare Ingredients: Place all the ingredients in the crockpot.

2. Cook: Cover and cook on low for 68 hours or on high for 34 hours.

3. Serve: Serve hot, garnished with fresh cilantro or avocado if desired.

Slow Cooker Tuscan Lentil Sloppy Joes

Try these Slow Cooker Tuscan Lentil Sloppy Joes for a twist on the classic recipe. This zero point dinner is hearty and healthy, perfect for a family meal.

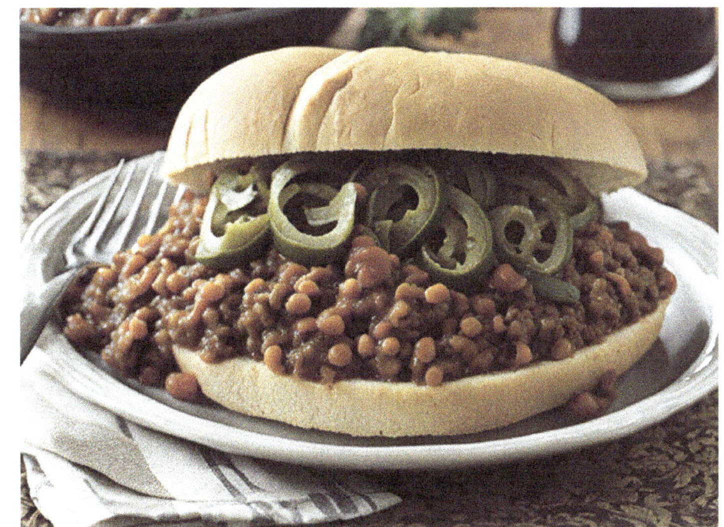

ingredients

- 1 cup lentils, rinsed
- 1 onion, diced
- 2 cloves garlic, minced
- 1 can diced tomatoes
- 1/4 cup tomato paste
- 1 tablespoon balsamic vinegar
- 1 teaspoon Italian seasoning
- 4 whole wheat buns (optional)
- Salt and pepper to taste

Preparation Time

68 hours

Cooking Time

68 hours

Serving Size

4

Nutrition (per serving)

- Protein: 12g
- Carbs: 35g
- Fat: 1g

Instructions

1. Prepare Ingredients: Place the lentils, onion, garlic, diced tomatoes, tomato paste, balsamic vinegar, Italian seasoning, salt, and pepper in the slow cooker.

2. Cook: Cover and cook on low for 68 hours or on high for 34 hours.

3. Serve: Serve the lentil mixture on whole wheat buns or over a bed of greens for a lowcarb option.

Cabbage Soup

Enjoy a comforting bowl of Cabbage Soup that's both hearty and nutritious. This recipe is perfect for a light yet satisfying dinner.

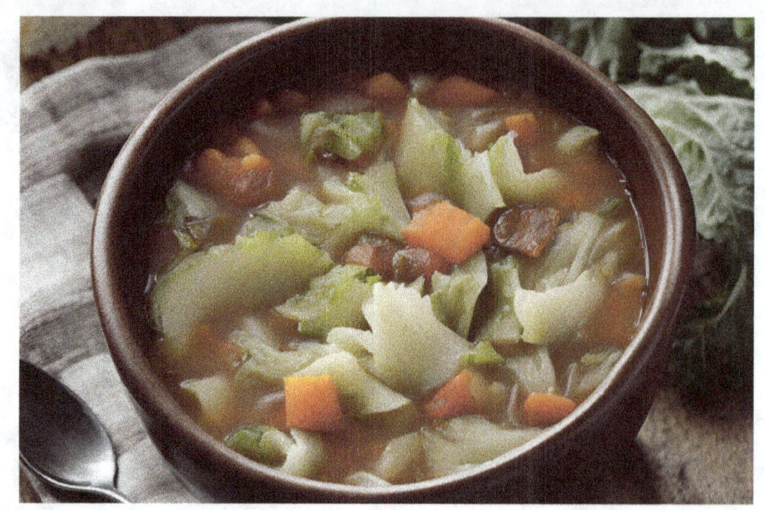

ingredients

- 1 small head of cabbage, chopped
- 1 large onion, diced
- 2 cloves garlic, minced
- 2 carrots, sliced
- 2 celery stalks, sliced
- 1 bell pepper, diced
- 1 can diced tomatoes
- 4 cups vegetable broth
- 1 teaspoon dried oregano
- 1 teaspoon dried basil
- Salt and pepper to taste

Preparation Time
45 minutes

Cooking Time
40 minutes

Serving Size
6

Nutrition (per serving)
- Protein: 2g
- Carbs: 10g
- Fat: 0g

Instructions

1. Prepare Vegetables: In a large pot, sauté the onion and garlic until softened.

2. Add Ingredients: Add the carrots, celery, bell pepper, cabbage, diced tomatoes, vegetable broth, oregano, basil, salt, and pepper.

3. Simmer: Bring to a boil, then reduce heat and simmer for 3040 minutes or until the vegetables are tender.

4. Serve: Serve hot, garnished with fresh parsley if desired.

Instant Pot Vegetarian Chili

This Instant Pot Vegetarian Chili is a quick and easy dinner option packed with flavor. It's a zero point meal that's perfect for a busy weeknight.

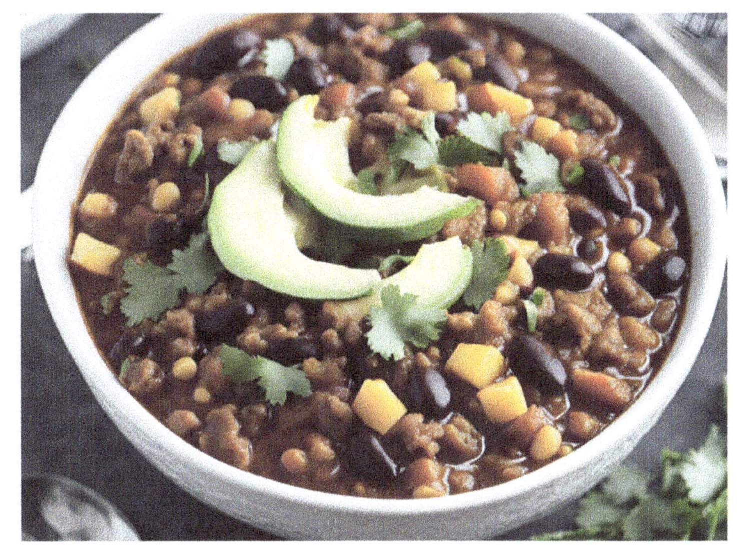

ingredients

- 1 cup dried lentils, rinsed
- 1 can black beans, rinsed and drained
- 1 can kidney beans, rinsed and drained
- 1 can diced tomatoes
- 1 onion, diced
- 1 bell pepper, diced
- 1 tablespoon chili powder
- 1 teaspoon cumin
- 4 cups vegetable broth
- Salt and pepper to taste
- 2 cloves garlic, minced

Preparation Time

30 minutes

Cooking Time

15 minutes

Serving Size

6

Nutrition (per serving)

- Protein: 12g
- Carbs: 30g
- Fat: 1g

Instructions

1. Prepare Ingredients: Add all ingredients to the Instant Pot.

2. Cook: Secure the lid and set the Instant Pot to high pressure for 15 minutes.

3. Release Pressure: Once cooking is complete, allow the pressure to release naturally for 10 minutes, then release any remaining pressure manually.

4. Serve: Serve hot, garnished with fresh cilantro or avocado if desired.

Skinny Bang Bang Shrimp

Indulge in these Skinny Bang Bang Shrimp for a delicious and guilt free dinner. This zero point recipe offers a healthier take on a restaurant favorite.

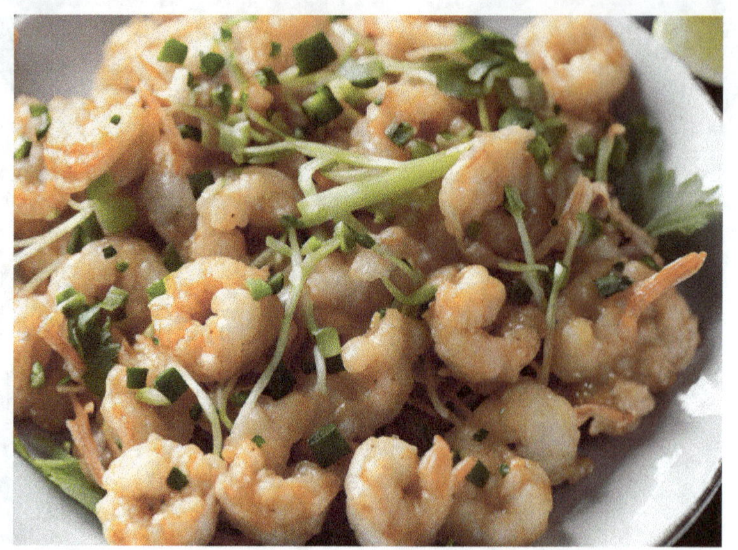

ingredients

- 1 pound shrimp, peeled and deveined
- 1/4 cup Greek yogurt
- 1 tablespoon hot sauce
- 1 teaspoon honey

- 1/2 teaspoon paprika
- Salt and pepper to taste
- Cooking spray
- 1/2 teaspoon garlic powder

Preparation Time
15 minutes

Cooking Time
6 minutes

Serving Size
4

Nutrition (per serving)
- Protein: 25g
- Carbs: 5g
- Fat: 2g

Instructions

1. Prepare Shrimp: In a bowl, mix Greek yogurt, hot sauce, honey, garlic powder, paprika, salt, and pepper. Add Shrimp and toss to coat.

2. Cook Shrimp: Heat a nonstick skillet over medium high heat and spray with cooking spray. Cook shrimp on each side for 23 minutes until opaque and cooked through.

3. Serve: Serve immediately, garnished with fresh cilantro if desired.

Grilled Shrimp Marinade with Shrimp Sauce

Enjoy a delicious and light dinner with this Grilled Shrimp Marinade with Shrimp Sauce. It's a flavorful meal that's perfect for a summer evening.

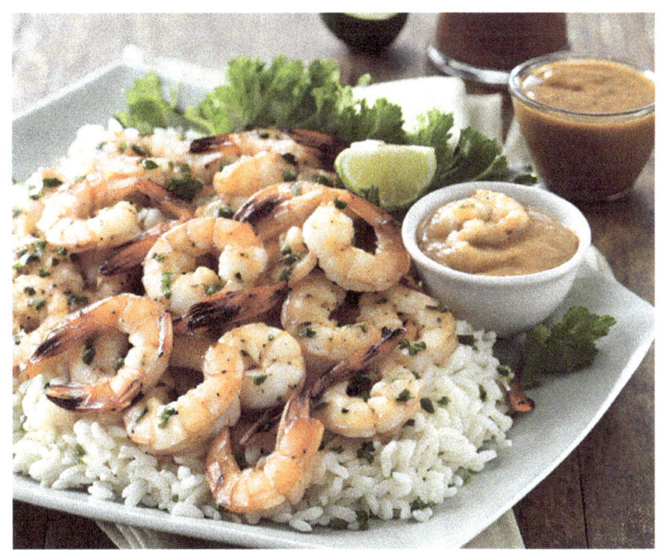

ingredients

- 1 pound shrimp, peeled and deveined
- Juice of 1 lemon
- 2 cloves garlic, minced
- 1 tablespoon olive oil
- 1 teaspoon dried oregano
- Salt and pepper to taste

Preparation Time

35 minutes

Cooking Time

6 minutes

Serving Size

4

Nutrition (per serving)

- Protein: 24g
- Carbs: 2g
- Fat: 3g

Instructions

1. Marinate Shrimp: In a bowl, mix lemon juice, garlic, olive oil, oregano, salt, and pepper. Add shrimp and marinate for at least 30 minutes.

2. Prepare Grill: Preheat grill to medium high heat.

3. Grill Shrimp: Thread shrimp onto skewers and grill for 23 minutes on each side until pink and cooked.

4. Serve: Serve immediately with grilled vegetables or a salad.

CHAPTER FIVE

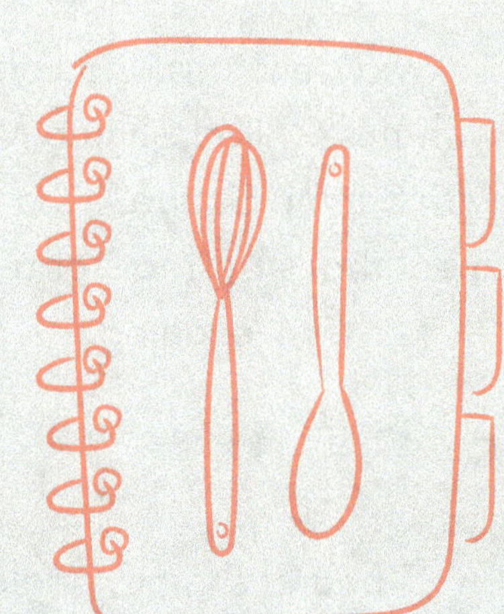

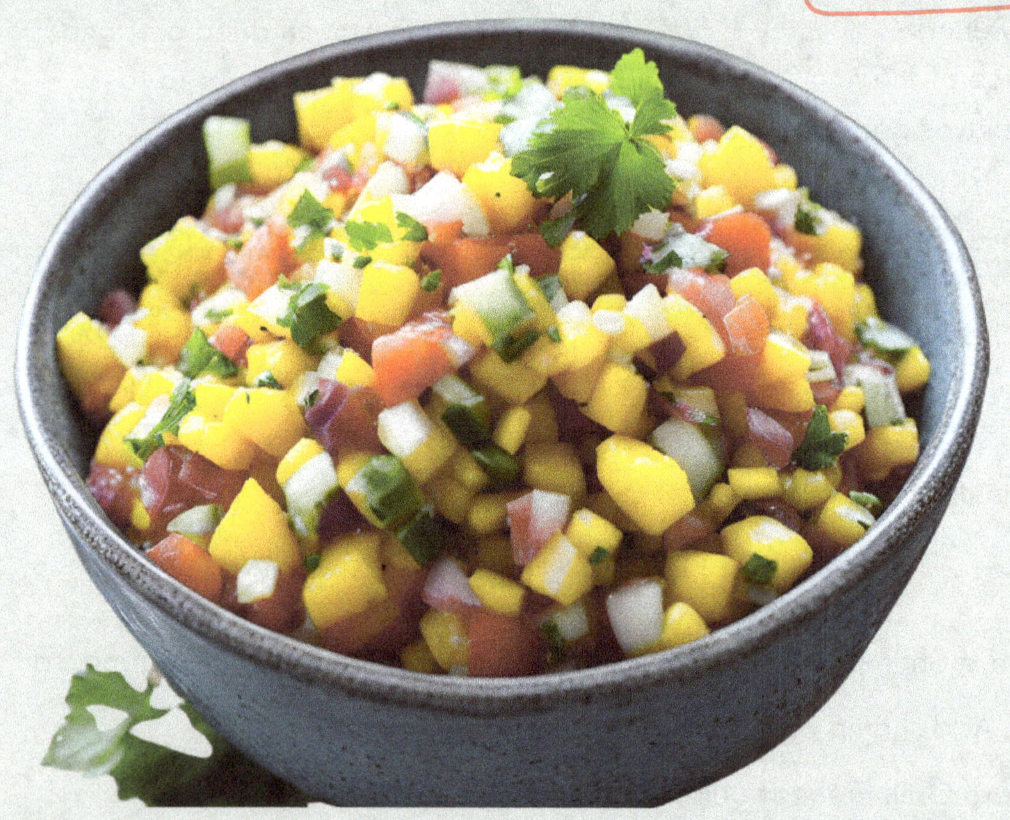

Dinner Recipes

Apple Slices with Cinnamon

Apple Slices with Cinnamon is a simple yet satisfying snack perfect for any time of the day. This zero point treat is delicious and packed with fiber and antioxidants.

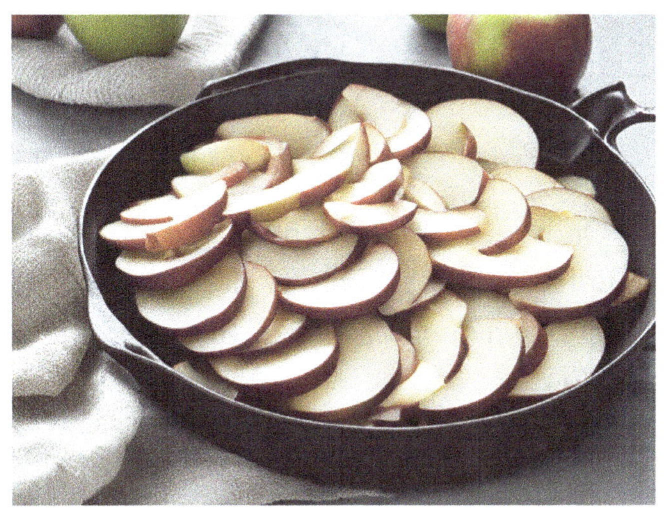

ingredients

- 1 apple, sliced
- 1/2 teaspoon ground cinnamon

Preparation Time

5 minutes

Serving Size

1

Nutrition (per serving)

- Protein: 0g
- Carbs: 21g
- Fat: 0g

Cooking Time

None

Instructions

1. Prepare Apple: Slice the apple into thin wedges.

2. Sprinkle Cinnamon: Sprinkle ground cinnamon over the apple slices.

3. Serve: Enjoy immediately.

Mixed Berry Sorbet

Indulge in a refreshing Mixed Berry Sorbet, perfect for cooling down on a warm day. This dessert is sweet, tangy, and incredibly easy to make.

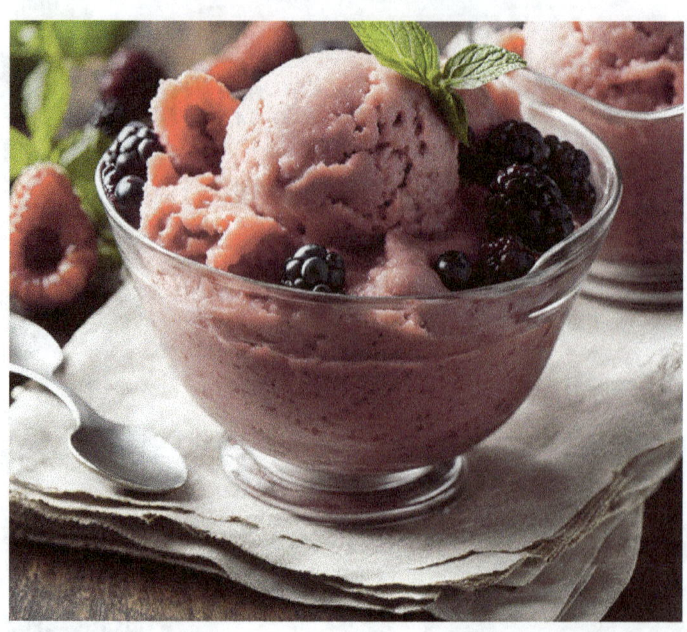

ingredients

- 2 cups mixed berries (strawberries, blueberries, raspberries, blackberries)
- 1 tablespoon lemon juice
- 1 tablespoon honey (optional)

Preparation Time
3 hours

Cooking Time
None

Serving Size
4

Nutrition (per serving)
- Protein: 1g
- Carbs: 12g
- Fat: 0g

Instructions

1. Blend Berries: In a blender or food processor, blend the mixed berries, lemon juice, and honey until smooth.

2. Freeze: Pour the mixture into a shallow dish and freeze for 23 hours, stirring every 30 minutes to break up any ice crystals.

3. Serve: Scoop into bowls and enjoy.

Carrot and Celery Sticks with Hummus

Carrot and Celery Sticks with Hummus make for a crunchy, nutritious, zero point snack. Perfect for a quick bite or a party appetizer, it's both healthy and satisfying.

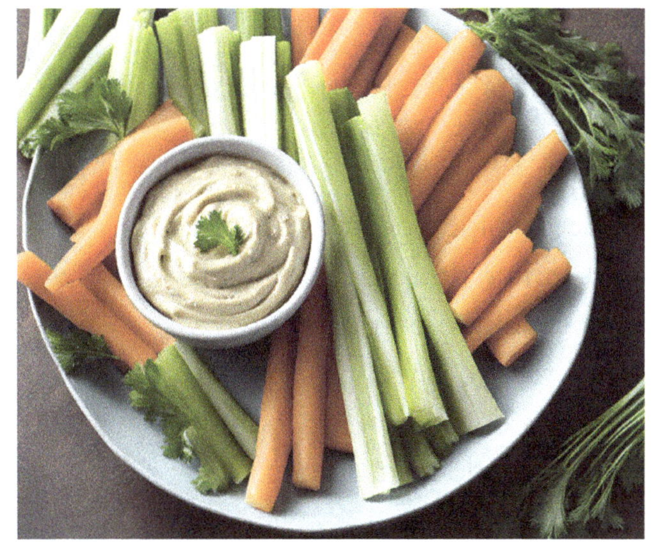

ingredients

- 2 carrots, cut into sticks
- 2 celery stalks, cut into sticks
- 1/2 cup homemade or store-bought zero point hummus

Preparation Time

10 minutes

Cooking Time

None

Serving Size

2

Nutrition (per serving)

- Protein: 2g
- Carbs: 15g
- Fat: 2g

Instructions

1. Prepare Vegetables: Cut the carrots and celery into sticks.

2. Serve with Hummus: Arrange the carrot and celery sticks on a plate with a serving of hummus.

3. Enjoy: Dip and enjoy!

Hard Boiled Eggs

Hardboiled eggs are a classic, protein packed snack that's simple to prepare. They're perfect for meal prepping and can be enjoyed independently or added to salads.

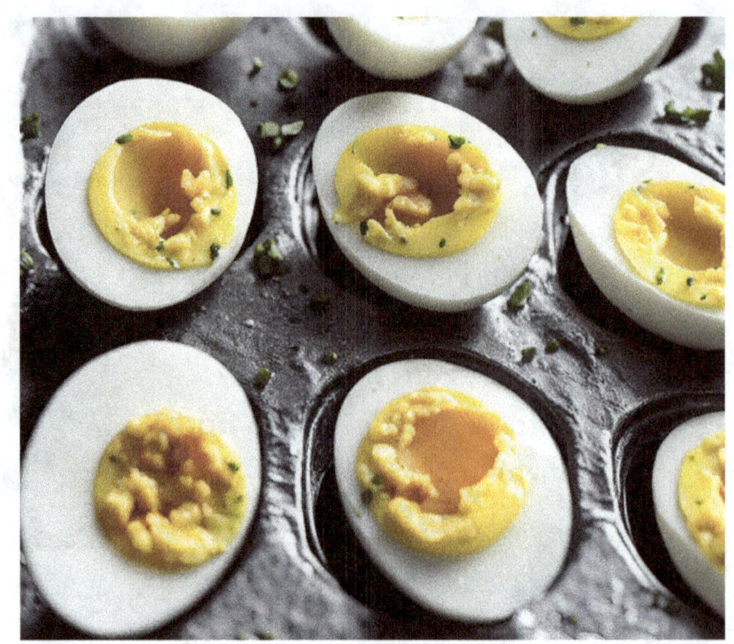

ingredients

- 4 large eggs

Preparation Time

15 minutes

Cooking Time

12 minutes

Serving Size

4

Nutrition (per serving)

- Protein: 6g
- Carbs: 1g
- Fat: 5g

Instructions

1. Boil Eggs: Place eggs in a pot and cover with water. Bring to a boil over medium high heat.

2. Cook Eggs: Once boiling, reduce heat and simmer for 912 minutes.

3. Cool Eggs: Transfer eggs to a bowl of ice water to cool for 5 minutes.

4. Peel and Serve: Peel the eggs and enjoy.

Cucumber Slices with Greek Yogurt Dip

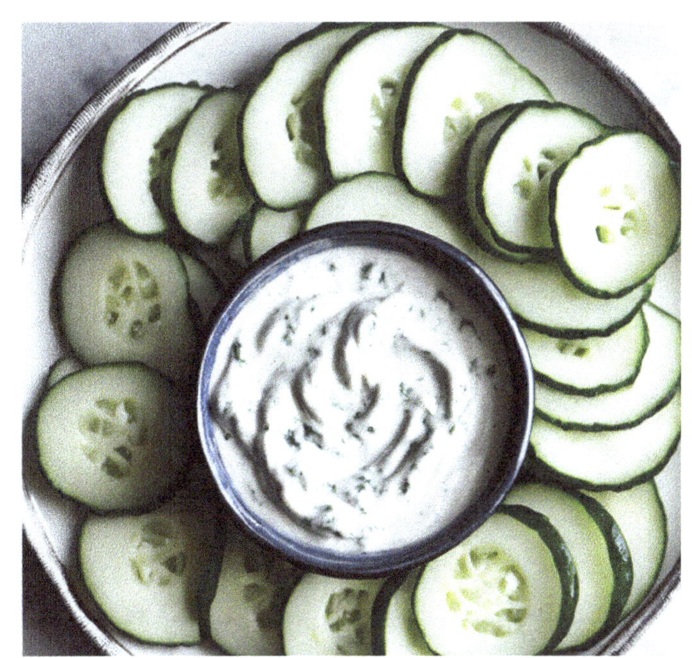

Cucumber Slices with Greek Yogurt Dip is a refreshing, creamy snack perfect for a healthy, zero point treat.

ingredients

- 1 cucumber, sliced
- 1/2 cup fat free Greek yogurt
- 1 teaspoon lemon juice
- 1 clove garlic, minced
- Salt and pepper to taste

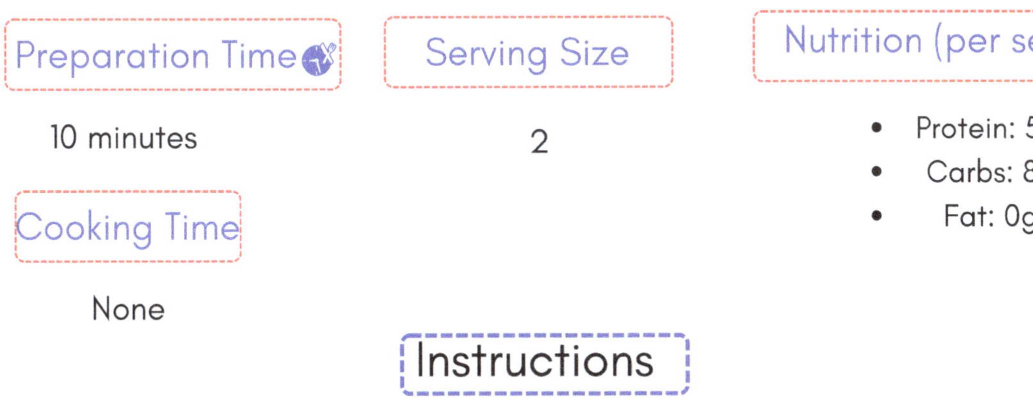

Preparation Time	Serving Size	Nutrition (per serving)
10 minutes	2	• Protein: 5g • Carbs: 8g • Fat: 0g

Cooking Time

None

Instructions

1. Prepare Dip: In a small bowl, mix Greek yogurt, lemon juice, garlic, salt, and pepper.

2. Slice Cucumber: Slice the cucumber into thin rounds.

3. Serve: Serve the cucumber slices with the Greek yogurt dip.

Frozen Fruit Pops

Cool off with these delicious Frozen Fruit Pops. They're easy to make, full of natural sweetness, and zero points.

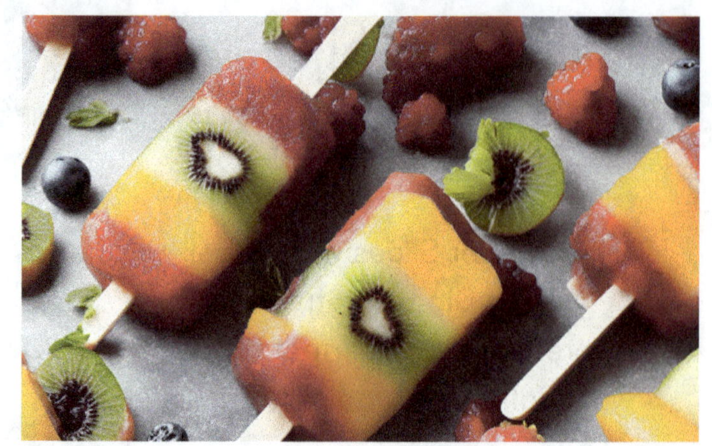

ingredients

- 2 cups mixed fruit (such as berries, mango, pineapple)
- 1 cup water
- 1 tablespoon honey (optional)

Preparation Time

4 hours

Cooking Time

None

Serving Size

4

Nutrition (per serving)

- Protein: 1g
- Carbs: 15g
- Fat: 0g

Instructions

1. Blend Ingredients: In a blender, blend the mixed fruit, water, and honey until smooth.

2. Pour into Molds: Pour the mixture into popsicle molds.

3. Freeze: Freeze for at least 4 hours or until solid.

4. Serve: Remove from molds and enjoy.

Spicy Roasted Cauliflower

Spicy Roasted Cauliflower is a flavorful and crunchy snack or side dish. It's a zero point recipe that's perfect for adding a little heat to your meal.

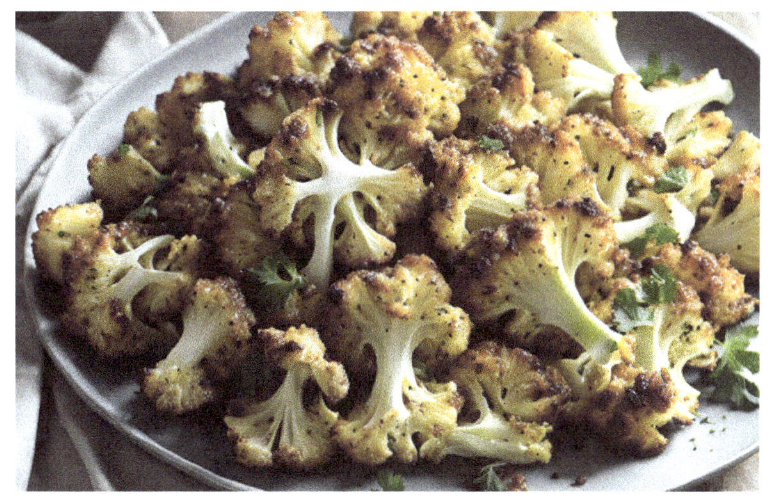

ingredients

- 1 head cauliflower, cut into florets
- 1 tablespoon olive oil
- 1 teaspoon paprika
- 1/2 teaspoon garlic powder
- 1/4 teaspoon cayenne pepper
- Salt and pepper to taste

Preparation Time

35 minutes

Cooking Time

25 minutes

Serving Size

4

Nutrition (per serving)

- Protein: 3g
- Carbs: 8g
- Fat: 3g

Instructions

1. Preheat Oven: Preheat your oven to 425°F (220°C).

2. Prepare Cauliflower: In a large bowl, toss the cauliflower florets with olive oil, paprika, garlic powder, cayenne pepper, salt, and pepper.

3. Roast: Spread the Cauliflower on a baking sheet and roast for 2530 minutes or until tender and golden brown.

4. Serve: Serve hot as a snack or side dish.

The Best 0Point Weight Watchers Cheesecake

Indulge in a creamy, delicious cheesecake without any guilt. This zero point Weight Watchers Cheesecake is a perfect dessert for those who want to satisfy their sweet tooth while sticking to their weight loss goals.

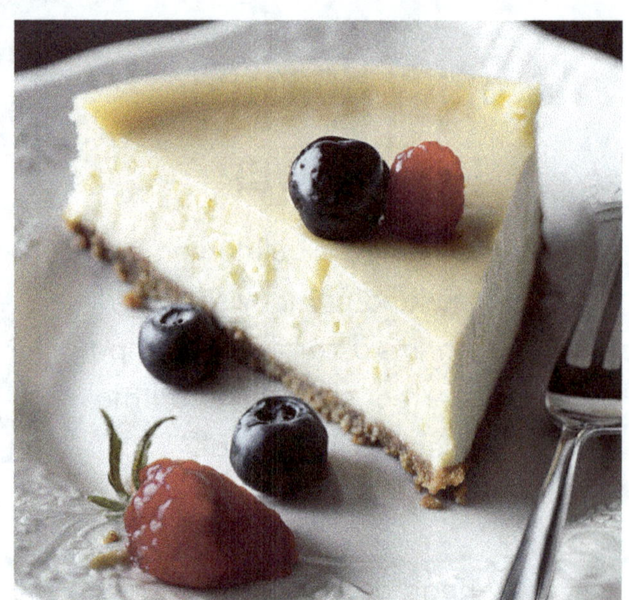

ingredients

- 3 cups fat free Greek yogurt
- 1 box sugar free, fat free cheesecake flavored pudding mix
- 3 eggs
- 1 teaspoon vanilla extract
- 2 tablespoons lemon juice

Preparation Time

5 hours

Cooking Time

30 minutes

Serving Size

8

Nutrition (per serving)

- Protein: 10g
- Carbs: 8g
- Fat: 0g

Instructions

1. Preheat Oven: Preheat your oven to 350°F (175°C).

2. Mix Ingredients: In a large bowl, combine the Greek yogurt, pudding mix, eggs, vanilla extract, and lemon juice. Mix until smooth.

3. Prepare Pan: Pour the mixture into a springform pan lined with parchment paper.

4. Bake: Bake for 30 minutes, then turn off the oven and let the cheesecake sit in the oven for another 30 minutes.

5. Chill: Refrigerate for at least 4 hours before serving.

Mango Corn Salsa

Add a burst of flavor to your meals with this refreshing Mango Corn Salsa. It's a zero point side dish perfect for summer BBQs or a topping for grilled chicken or fish.

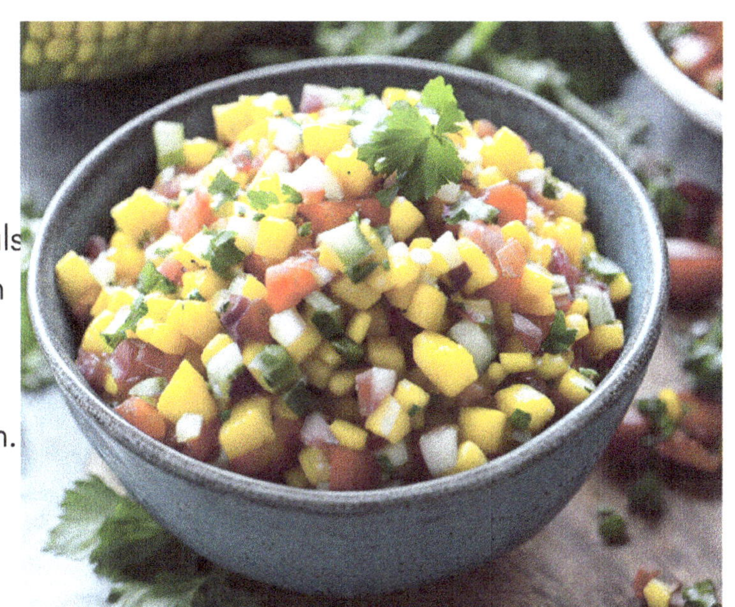

ingredients

- 1 cup diced mango
- 1 cup corn kernels
- 1/4 cup diced red onion
- 1/4 cup chopped cilantro
- 1 jalapeño, seeded and diced
- Juice of 1 lime
- Salt and pepper to taste

Preparation Time

10 minutes

Cooking Time

None

Serving Size

4

Nutrition (per serving)

- Protein: 1g
- Carbs: 12g
- Fat: 0g

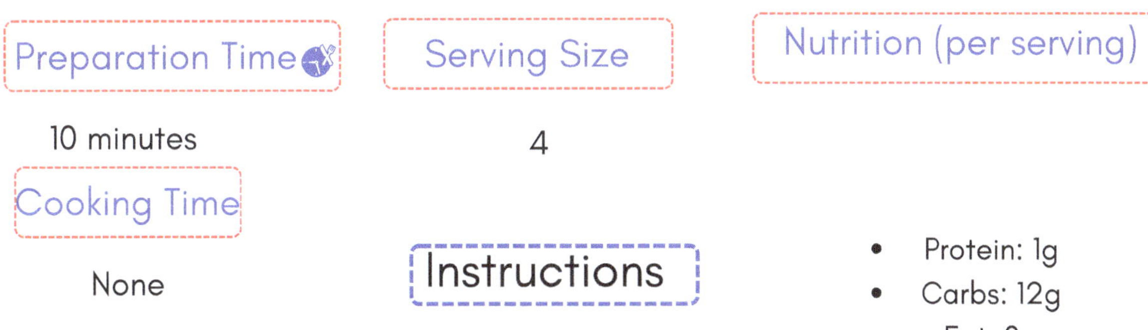

Instructions

1. Prepare Ingredients: In a large bowl, combine the diced mango, corn, red onion, cilantro, and jalapeño.

2. Add Lime Juice: Squeeze the lime juice over the salsa and season with salt and pepper.

3. Mix and Serve: Mix well and serve immediately or refrigerate until ready to use.

Slow Cooker Spaghetti Squash

This Slow Cooker Spaghetti Squash offers a lowcarb, zero point alternatives to pasta. It's a simple, healthy side dish that pairs perfectly with your favorite marinara sauce.

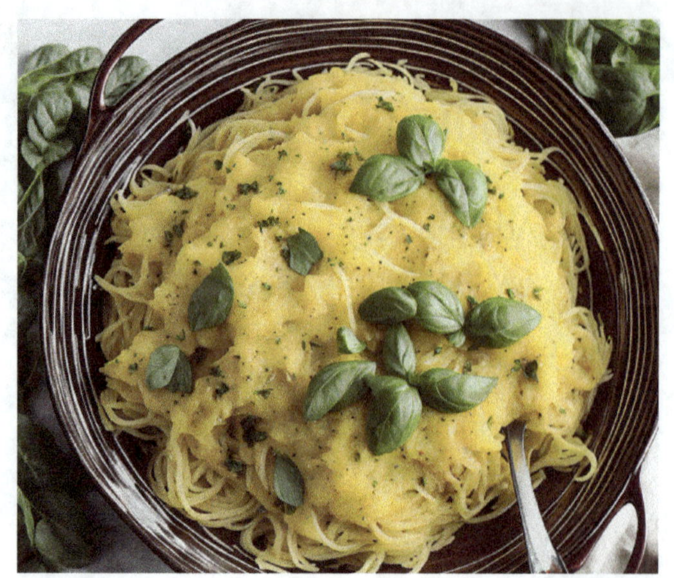

ingredients

- 1 spaghetti squash
- 1 cup water

Preparation Time

46 hours

Cooking Time

46 hours

Serving Size

4

Nutrition (per serving)

- Protein: 1g
- Carbs: 7g
- Fat: 0g

Instructions

1. Prepare Squash: Cut the spaghetti squash in half and remove the seeds.

2. Add Water: Pour the water into the slow cooker and place the squash halves cut side down.

3. Cook: Cover and cook on low for 46 hours or until the Squash is tender.

4. Shred Squash: Use a fork to scrape out the spaghetti like strands and serve with your favorite sauce.

Slow Cooker Tomato Sauce

Make your flavorful tomato sauce with this easy Slow Cooker Tomato Sauce recipe. It's a zero point sauce that's perfect for pasta, pizza, or as a dipping sauce.

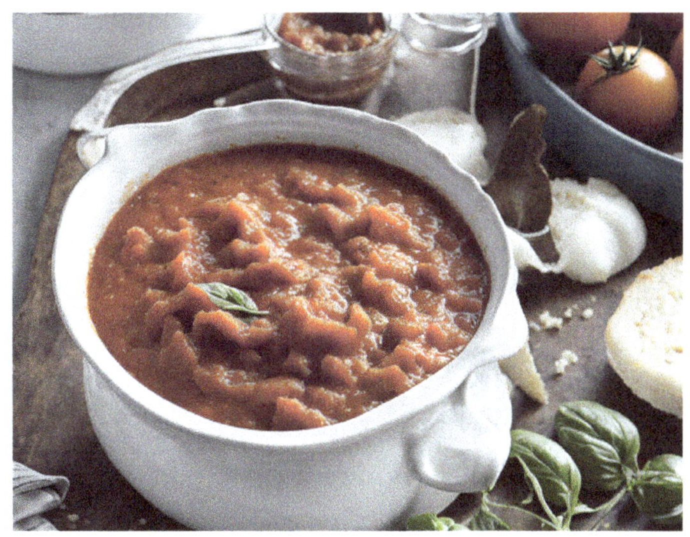

ingredients

- 2 cans whole peeled tomatoes
- 1 onion, diced
- 2 cloves garlic, minced
- 1 teaspoon dried oregano
- 1 teaspoon dried basil
- Salt and pepper to taste
-

Preparation Time

68 hours

Cooking Time

68 hours

Serving Size

6

Nutrition (per serving)

- Protein: 2g
- Carbs: 10g
- Fat: 0g

Instructions

1. Prepare Ingredients: Add the tomatoes, onion, garlic, oregano, basil, salt, and pepper to the slow cooker.

2. Cook: Cover and cook on low for 68 hours, or until the sauce has thickened and the flavors have melded together.

3. Blend: An immersion blender blends the sauce until smooth.

4. Serve: Serve hot or store in the refrigerator for up to a week.

Smiley's Famous Zero Point B.B.Q. Sauce

Add a tangy and smoky flavor to your meals with Smiley's Famous Zero Point B.B.Q. Sauce. This homemade sauce is perfect for grilling and adds a delicious touch to any dish.

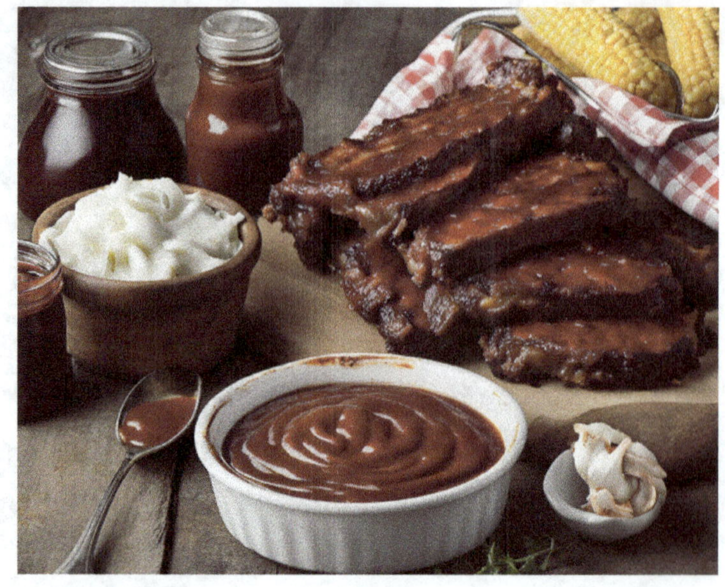

ingredients

- 1 cans tomato paste
- 1/2 cup apple cider vinegar
- 1/4 cup Worcestershire sauce
- 1/4 cup yellow mustard
- 1/4 cup sugar free sweetener
- 1 teaspoon smoked paprika
- 1 teaspoon garlic powder
- 1 teaspoon onion powder
- Salt and pepper to taste

Preparation Time

25 minutes

Cooking Time

20 minutes

Serving Size

10

Nutrition (per serving)

- Protein: 0g
- Carbs: 2g
- Fat: 0g

Instructions

1. Mix Ingredients: In a saucepan, combine the tomato paste, apple cider vinegar, Worcestershire sauce, yellow mustard, sweetener, smoked paprika, garlic powder, onion powder, salt, and pepper.

2. Cook: Bring to a boil over medium heat, then reduce heat and simmer for 20 minutes, stirring occasionally.

3. Serve: Serve hot or store in the refrigerator for up to a week.

A Note of Thanks

Thank you for choosing the Zero Point Weight Loss Recipes Cookbook as your guide on this journey. Your commitment to improving your health and wellbeing is truly commendable. We hope these recipes have provided delicious and nutritious options that make healthy eating easy and enjoyable.

We Value Your Feedback

Your feedback is precious to us. We would love to hear about your experiences with the cookbook. What recipes did you enjoy the most? How has this book helped you on your weight loss journey? Your reviews and comments help us to continue improving and providing valuable resources to our readers.

Please take a moment to leave a review or share your thoughts online. Your insights can help others who are embarking on their health journeys.

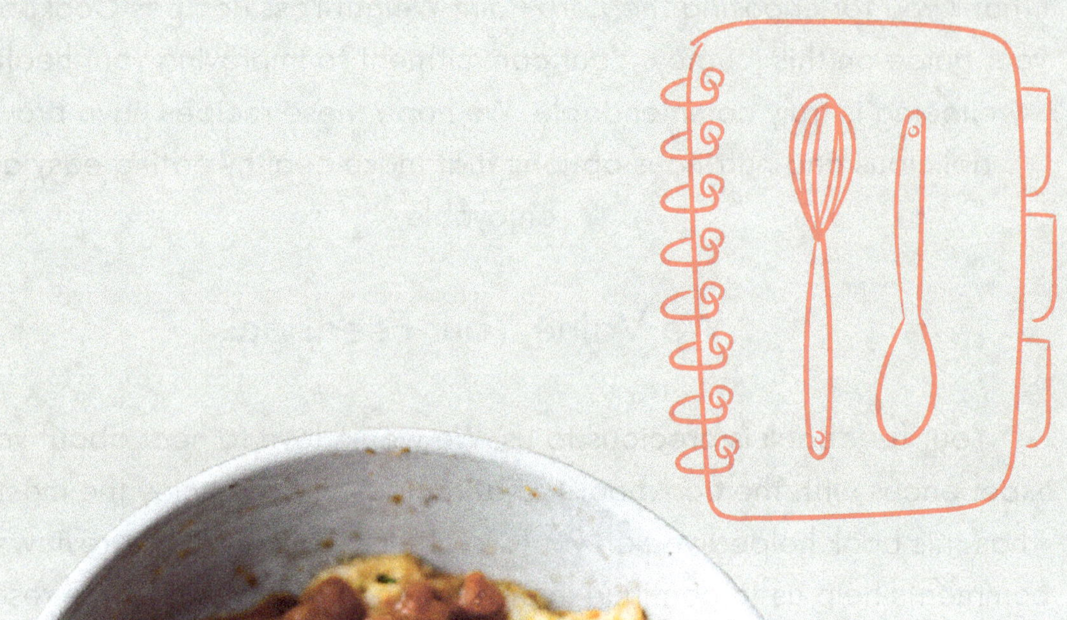

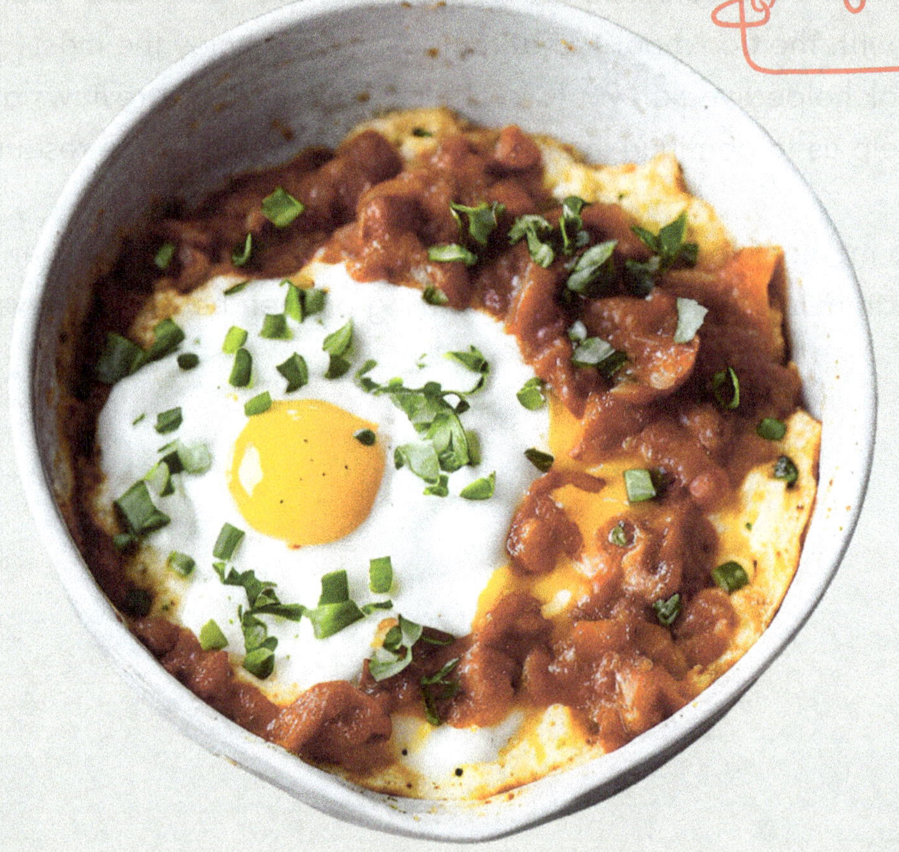

BONUS

MEAL PLAN

DAY 1	DAY 2
Breakfast: Veggie Omelets Lunch: Grilled Chicken Salad Dinner: Baked Salmon with Asparagus Snack: Apple Slices with Cinnamon	Breakfast: Fruit and Yogurt Parfait Lunch: Turkey Lettuce Wraps Dinner: Zucchini Noodles with Marinara Sauce Snack: Carrot and Celery Sticks with Hummus

DAY 3	DAY 4
Breakfast: Spinach and Mushroom Scramble Lunch: Quinoa and Black Bean Salad Dinner: Chicken and Vegetable Skewers Snack: HardBoiled Eggs	Breakfast: Banana Pancakes Lunch: Cucumber and Tomato Salad Dinner: Stuffed Bell Peppers Snack: Cucumber Slices with Greek Yogurt Dip

DAY 5	DAY 6
Breakfast: Berry Smoothie Bowl Lunch: Chipotle Chicken Casserole Dinner: Cauliflower Fried Rice Snack: Frozen Fruit Pops	Breakfast: Apple Pie Parfait Lunch: Grilled Crab Legs Dinner: Slow Cooker Tomato Balsamic Chicken Snack: Spicy Roasted Cauliflower

DAY 7	DAY 8
Breakfast: 4Ingredient Microwave Mug Frittata Lunch: Vegetable StirFry Dinner: Turkey, Corn, and Black Bean Chili Snack: Jello Grapes	Breakfast: Salmon Omelet in a Mug Lunch: Egg Salad Dinner: Lentil Soup Snack: Mixed Berry Sorbet

MEAL PLAN

DAY 9	DAY 10
Breakfast: Skinny Western Omelet Muffins Lunch: One Pan of Chicken Fajitas Dinner: Garden Vegetable Soup Snack: Carrot and Celery Sticks with Hummus	Breakfast: Kodiak Cake Muffins Lunch: Grilled Chicken Salad Dinner: Crockpot Bean Soup Snack: HardBoiled Eggs
DAY 11	DAY 12
Breakfast: Cheesy Ham and Egg Cups Lunch: Turkey Lettuce Wraps Dinner: Slow Cooker Tuscan Lentil Sloppy Joes Snack: Apple Slices with Cinnamon	Breakfast: WW Crepes Lunch: Cucumber and Tomato Salad Dinner: Chicken Enchilada Stuffed Zucchini Snack: Cucumber Slices with Greek Yogurt Dip
DAY 13	DAY 14
Breakfast: Veggie Omelette Lunch: Quinoa and Black Bean Salad Dinner: Instant Pot Vegetarian Chili Snack: Mixed Berry Sorbet	Breakfast: Fruit and Yogurt Parfait Lunch: Egg Salad Dinner: Skinny Bang Bang Shrimp Snack: Jello Grapes
DAY 15	DAY 16
Breakfast: Spinach and Mushroom Scramble Lunch: Vegetable StirFry Dinner: Baked Salmon with Asparagus Snack: Spicy Roasted Cauliflower	Breakfast: Banana Pancakes Lunch: Chipotle Chicken Casserole Dinner: Grilled Shrimp Marinade with Shrimp Sauce Snack: Carrot and Celery Sticks with Hummus

MEAL PLAN

DAY 17	DAY 18
Breakfast: Berry Smoothie Bowl Lunch: Grilled Crab Legs Dinner: Cauliflower Fried Rice Snack: Frozen Fruit Pops	Breakfast: Apple Pie Parfait Lunch: Turkey Lettuce Wraps Dinner: Slow Cooker Tomato Balsamic Chicken Snack: HardBoiled Eggs
DAY 19	**DAY 20**
Breakfast: 4Ingredient Microwave Mug Frittata Lunch: Quinoa and Black Bean Salad Dinner: Turkey, Corn, and Black Bean Chili Snack: Apple Slices with Cinnamon	Breakfast: Salmon Omelet in a Mug Lunch: Cucumber and Tomato Salad Dinner: Slow Cooker Tuscan Lentil Sloppy Joes Snack: Mixed Berry Sorbet
DAY 21	**DAY 22**

Conclusion

As you end the Zero Point Weight Loss Recipes Cookbook, it's essential to reflect on the journey you've undertaken. Embracing a healthier lifestyle through zero point foods is a significant step towards better health and wellbeing. This cookbook has provided many delicious, nutritious recipes to make your weight loss journey enjoyable and sustainable.

Encouragement and Motivation

1. Celebrate Your Achievements: Every healthy meal you prepare and enjoy is a step towards a healthier you. Celebrate your successes, no matter how small they may seem. Each one is a milestone on your journey.
2. Stay Motivated: Remember why you started this journey. Keep that motivation in mind, whether it's to feel better, improve your health, or achieve a specific weight loss goal. Use it to drive you forward, especially when staying on track is challenging.
3. Consistency is Key: Your changes today will impact your health. Stick with the habits you've built through these recipes. Consistency in your eating patterns will yield longterm results.
4. Enjoy the Process: Cooking and eating should be enjoyable experiences. Take pleasure in discovering new recipes, flavors, and cooking techniques. Share your culinary creations with friends and family, and relish the joy that good food brings.
5. Keep Learning and adapting: The journey to health is ongoing. Explore new recipes, adapt to changing tastes, and stay informed about nutrition. Your body and your health will thank you.